THE SCHIZOPHRENIC CHILD

A PRIMER FOR PARENTS AND PROFESSIONALS

DR. SHEILA CANTOR

WITH A PREFACE BY DR. PETER TANGUAY

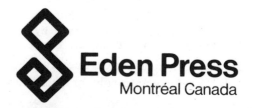

Eden Press
Montréal Canada

THE SCHIZOPHRENIC CHILD
A Primer for Parents and Professionals
by
Dr. Sheila Cantor

© 1982 Eden Press Incorporated
Montreal, Quebec, Canada
and
St. Albans, Vermont, U.S.A.

ISBN: 0-920792-13-8
First Edition

Credits:
Cover Design: J.W. Stewart
Cover Photograph: Peter Lowery
Child Model: Jess Dutton
Typesetting & Production:
Vicky Bach and Molly Pulver, Hamilton, Ontario

Printed and bound in Canada by
T. H. Best Printing Company Limited
Dépôt légal - deuxième trimestre 1982
Bibliothèque nationale du Québec

THE
SCHIZOPHRENIC
CHILD

TO

Drs. Lauretta Bender
         and
Barbara Fish

Without whose pioneering work this book
could not have been written.

TABLE OF CONTENTS

Author's Note

This book was written in the *International Year of the Disabled Person*. In Manitoba at least, the Schizophrenia Treatment and Research Foundation was invited and welcomed as a regular participant in all events which commemorated this special year. We have dared to hope that the time is here, at last, when society can view schizophrenia as a disabler which deserves the same compassion and level of care as any other disease process. We have dared to hope that we are finally ready to welcome the mentally ill back into our communities.

Integration will take time. Support systems will have to be set in place which will address themselves to the needs of the chronic schizophrenic. Only then will it become possible for the chronic schizophrenic to not only live in the community but to make a contribution to that community.

My deepest thanks are due to those who have taken time to read this manuscript and make the suggestions which have improved the text, Mrs. Leona Lakser, Mr. Russell Dueck, Mr. Tom Roche, Drs. Prosen, Snyder, McRae, and de von Flindt. The support and encouragement of my chairman, Dr. Harry Prosen, and my good friend Dr. Peter Tanguay, are gratefully acknowledged. A special thanks to my secretary, Mrs. Brenda Tyre, who required the patience of Job to keep typing and retyping the manuscript.

i

Most of all, it was for my own patients and for their families that this book was undertaken. Their courage and coping capacity were constant sources of inspiration. It was they who tested every suggested intervention and who were always my greatest teachers. The services which they so urgently require are not yet available here in Manitoba. Together, however, "we shall overcome."

Sheila Cantor
Winnipeg, Manitoba
August 1981

The research upon which this book was based has been generously supported by the White Cross Guild Trust Fund (Grant # 387-3137-18) and the Lions' Disability Fund (Grant # 387-3137-18).

PREFACE

There was a time, a few years ago, when I knew a great deal about childhood psychoses. I had received from Leo Kanner's writings the precise picture of early infantile autism, and I understood from the classic papers of Michael Rutter and Israel Kolvin about "early onset psychosis" and "late onset psychosis". "Early onset psychosis" was diagnosable prior to age three, while "late onset psychosis" was rarely seen prior to age seven or eight, and was not usually preceded by any severe disturbances in relating, cognition or language. There was of course Lauretta Bender's "childhood schizophrenia", but if in fact there were but two distinct forms of psychosis in children, and "late onset psychosis" was the downward extension (and not too far downward at that) of adult schizophrenia, then why not allow "childhood schizophrenia" to find its rightful place in the graveyard of historical terminology, to lie alongside such other heavies as symbiotic psychosis, atypical ego development, and dementia praecox? And, then, of course there came DSM-III. Its message was clear: there is but one schizophrenia, and DSM-III is its prophet. Yes, life was simple and uncomplicated, and the way was clear to get on with more serious work.

In 1977 the National Institute of Mental Health funded the UCLA Child Psychiatry Clinical Research Center whose goals were to study the etiology, prevention, and treatment not only of early infantile autism, but of all forms of psychosis in childhood. Over the past few years the Center has grown from some five projects (all studying autistic children) to some 25 projects investigating important questions in psychotic children whose ages range from two to twelve years. What my many colleagues and I have learned over the past few years has led me to realize how incomplete was my knowledge about childhood psychosis before the Center began.

From the recent literature, and from work done in our Center, it seems reasonable to suggest that early infantile autism is in a sense a man-made syndrome, useful perhaps for shorthand communication of a clinical picture between mental health professionals or educators, but not a syndrome having a unitary cause or even a unitary symptomatology. Looking at children who fit the DSM-III category of "pervasive developmental difficulties", one sees individuals whose symptoms range from classically autistic to less and less "autistic" until we reach those who are simply mentally retarded without features of autism, or who have serious disorders of communication with relatively little disturbance in relating to others. It would also appear that in those few instances where factors have been identified as important to the development of the syndrome of autism (e.g. inborn errors of metabolism, brain degenerative diseases, encephalitis), they are the very same ones which lead to non-autistic forms of mental retardation and developmental disability. Perhaps it is not any one specific factor or set of factors which is critical, but the time at which the factors exert their pathological influences upon the developing brain.

But if I have come to understand early infantile autism from a somewhat different perspective, my understanding of "childhood schizophrenia" has been even more radically adjusted. These children do exist, not only in the "late onset childhood psychosis" form described by Rutter and by Kolvin, but in the form described by Lauretta Bender and Barbara Fish. Nor are the prodromal features of the disorder uniform between children. Some of our children are described as having been relatively normal until age four or five years (with perhaps a mild delay in their language acquisition), while others were diagnosed as autistic or "atypically autistic" by our clinic faculty or by others when they were initially seen at age three or four years.

These children are not necessarily found in psychiatric clinics (especially ones whose staff does not believe they exist), but are much in evidence in special education classrooms, psychiatric residential centers for children who cannot be maintained at home, in day-schools for the emotionally disturbed, and in State and Provincial hospitals. From a diagnostic viewpoint it may be difficult to fit these children into the DSM-III category of schizophrenia (not surprising since the diagnostic criteria were developed for use with adults who have quite different language and cognitive abilities in comparison to children), though they may sometimes fit into the category "Psychotic Disorders Not Elsewhere Classified" under the diagnosis of schizophreniform psychosis or atypical psychosis. Failing this, it may always be possible to classify the children on Axis 2 as schizotypal personality disorder. I had occasion recently to review the monograph "Psychopathological Disorders in Childhood: Theoretical Considerations and a Proposed Classification" published in 1966 by the Group for the Advancement of Psychiatry. Within the proposed classification there was, under the label of "childhood schizophrenia", a very good description of these children. It would appear that for the past decade or so some of us had "lost" these children, so to speak, and are now only rediscovering them once more.

I doubt that our experiences in the Clinical Research Center are unique, and I expect that we will soon see a major resurgence of interest in childhood schizophrenia and in schizophrenic children. Sheila Cantor's book comes at a most opportune moment. Dr. Cantor is an extremely hard worker (she is a sort of one-person clinical research center), she is an acutely perceptive clinician, a creative research investigator, and she obviously cares very much for the children. Her description of the schizophrenic children and their development in the present book is one of the most complete which has appeared to date. It is the picture which has emerged from her own observations and research work. There are some who may object to what they see as the rather unambiguous manner in which the facts are presented, or to what they may feel are per-haps over-generalizations, but no matter: Dr. Cantor has painted a well-defined and relatively comprehensive picture of the schizophrenic child, and now it is up to others to come up with evidence to disprove what she states, or to modify it with observations and data which they themselves develop.

There is another aspect to this book which merits particular attention, and that is the notice which the author gives to the political aspects of childhood schizo-phrenia. An analogy can be drawn between what she perceives to be an unmet need in childhood schizophrenia with the plight of autistic children prior to the founding of the National Society for Autistic Children. Until that time, parents of autistic children had relatively little means to force school systems to provide schooling for their chil-dren, nor to lead reluctant mental health services admin-istrators to give their children access to the special programs available to retarded and other handicapped children. NSAC not only has given the parents of autistic children the means effectively to make their collective voices heard, but it has provided the opportunity for the parents themselves to develop innovative and creative programs for their children including respite care services, weekend and summer recreation programs, and a special residential program for adolescent autistic persons.

No such organization exists for schizophrenic children. Dr. Cantor's call for schizophrenic children and their parents to come "out of the closet" is an ambitious one, demanding much work from those who heed her advice. Recently, Dr. Cantor herself has spearheaded the development of an organization for the parents of schizophrenic children in Manitoba, a move which has profound implications for the general welfare of all schizophrenic children.

May this book mark the start of a new era! May it help focus our attention on a population of children who have been neglected by many child psychiatrists in the past decade, and may it lead to the development of new and better methods of treatment.

Peter Tanguay, M.D., Professor in Child Psychiatry, Director, Division of Child Psychiatry, Clinical Research Centre, U.C.L.A. — Neuropsychiatric Institute, Los Angeles, California

"I HAVE A SON . . . "

by Janine Stuart

"I HAVE A SON . . ."
by Janine Stuart

Eleven years have passed since I gave birth to my son Jason. I can remember the first moment that I held Jason in my arms, and all the love in my heart poured out to him. He looked so perfect to me.

As time passed, it became evident that he was not so perfect. There was something definitely wrong. I never knew what to observe in a child to detect any problems a baby might have emotionally. He appeared to be a content baby, and never too demanding. He sat up by himself at six months old, and started to walk at fourteen months. Fourteen months is a little slow to start walking, but not so slow that it would be considered a problem. When he was a year old he was not speaking a single word. He was a very hyperactive child. He would bounce on the bed for hours at a time, and when he wasn't bouncing, he would be spinning objects on the floor. The nights were long, as he never seemed to require much sleep. I would have to rock him, and walk with him in my arms to try to relax him. It would last until five in the morning, and then finally he would give in to sleep.

A year went by, and Jason still was not talking. Someone had suggested that I take him to a nursery school where he could communicate with other children. A doctor would give each child a complete examination

1

before they were allowed to attend this particular nursery. I was called in to meet the doctor, and discuss the results of Jason's tests. She said that Jason had the general appearance of a mongoloid. She then went on to say that although he had the appearance of one, the tests proved negative. She left me with the feeling that something was definitely wrong with him, but I still did not know what.

My next step was to bring him to our pediatrician. I explained to him what the other doctor had stated. He reassured me that there was nothing about Jason that would lead him to believe that Jason had Down's Syndrome (the old term is mongolism). He was not overly concerned about Jason's speechlessness either. He said that children develop at their own speed. He suggested that if I was still concerned, he could refer me to a child psychologist. I took the referral, and knew we were heading in the right direction.

We went to the Child Development Clinic, and the psychologist there observed Jason. He was put through basic tests of stacking blocks, drawing lines, etc. He showed little interest and was trying desperately to escape the office. We discussed Jason's behaviour at home. I told her how he jumped on the bed for hours, and how he enjoyed being alone in a room playing records and watching them spin. I also mentioned how he would giggle spontaneously for no apparent reason. Her diagnosis was that Jason was autistic. She went on to explain what autism was, and Jason certainly fit the description. I did not want to believe this, but it was quite evident. I left the doctor's office with the feeling of complete grief and dismay.

I knew that no matter how upset I was, or how grim the future looked, I could not give up. I loved Jason too much and I would be of no use to him if I were to drown in my own self-pity. I very seldom left him alone, trying not to give in to his desire to be in solitude. I am not claiming that my methods were of any benefit, but at the time, it seemed like the right thing to do. I would hold and kiss him, and tell him over and over again that I loved him. It really hurts when you pour all your emotions into someone you love so much, and don't get any feedback. He never gave me any eye contact. I would hold his head and ask him to look at me, his eyes would look everywhere but not into mine.

As Jason grew older he developed different fears. He was frightened of television commercials, not all of them, but certain ones. He would scream and cry for hours. If someone on television broke something, he would go completely wild and start breaking things around the house. One night he woke up in a fit of terror. He was screaming and I ran to his crib to pick him up. I tried to comfort him, but his body completely stiffened up and he seemed to hate my touch. He was fighting his way out of my arms, kicking and biting me. I held onto him and was very frightened. I realized how very disturbed my son was.

I had tried different methods to modify his behaviour. One was isolating him in a room for five minutes. The psychologist had suggested trying that as punishment. Unfortunately, it never worked. He would break the bedroom windows with his head. I felt so strongly that he could not control these fits, and did feel guilty for punishing him. These times were very hard on me emotionally and physically. It was a constant battle to get Jason to sleep at night, and to keep him happy during the day.

Jason was only interested in inanimate objects. He would spend a great deal of time with a magnetic alphabet board. One evening he started spelling words on it— "hot", "cold", "yes", "no", "mother", "root beer". I sat there astounded. To follow up my curiosity, I purposely misspelled words—he corrected them. From that moment on I knew he had the potential to learn. He was only three years old, he was not talking but he was spelling. I thought I would use his interest in the alphabet to my advantage. I cut out pictures of our family, and along side each of them, I printed their names. He watched with great interest, and after weeks of going over them, and saying the names aloud, he started saying them with me. It was so fascinating to hear him speak, I never imagined him ever talking.

Jason had been attending a half day programme at the Society for Crippled Children and Adults. They had tried to toilet train him there, but were unable to. The only benefit from this programme I felt, was that it enabled me to have a rest from Jason.

When he was four years old he was transferred to a full day programme at the St. Amant Centre for retarded children. I had mixed feelings about letting him attend this programme. Jason was not retarded, and even though I was fearful that this would do more harm than good, it was the only facility available. When Jason turned six, there was an alternate programme available at the Health Sciences Centre. This programme was more suitable to his needs. The children there were much the same as Jason. There was a remarkable improvement in Jason during his time in this programme. After one year there, they did a complete analysis on Jason's academic abilities. At seven he was functioning at a twelve year old level in some academic subjects. He could read virtually anything. Between the ages of six and eight he came a long way. I was almost ready to believe he would outgrow this disorder. It was a nice thought, but unfortunately not a reality.

When Jason was eight Dr. Sheila Cantor became the new Director of the Day Treatment Programme. Once again there was a new psychiatrist for Jason, and a new label. She told me Jason was schizophrenic. I had the misconception that schizophrenia was a split personality, and that a large majority of them were psychotic killers. The media would lead one to believe that the assumption was correct. Dr. Cantor went on to explain the nature of schizophrenia. I listened, but I was still not convinced that Jason was suffering from this disorder.

Every time a different diagnosis was made, I had to face another type of acceptance. I was very frustrated because every doctor had a different label for Jason. I was beginning to lose complete faith in the psychiatric field. It seemed to amount to only guess work on the doctors' part.

I met with Dr. Cantor on many occasions, and the more I learned about the disease, the more Jason fit into that category. It was the only diagnosis that I could say was "right on".*

As the years have passed, Jason has changed. He has improved remarkably. He is a very warm, loving child. Every night when I walk by his bedroom, he says "I love you mommy". It makes all the pains of the past seem so

---

*Dr. Michael Rutter saw this child at age eight and a half and confirmed the diagnosis of "Childhood Schizophrenia"—despite the child's early age of onset. Dr. Rutter is an advocate of the viewpoint that psychosis with onset prior to the age of 30 months has no relationship to schizophrenia.[1]

worthwhile. When he was young, I had thought of placing him in an institution. The thought would tear me apart, but at the time it seemed like the only solution. They were very difficult times for me. I felt physically and mentally exhausted. However, I am happy with my decision to keep him with me; and it has definitely paid off.

I am still very worried about his future and how he will survive. Without proper facilities for treatment and research available, his future does not seem too bright. I know he has a lot of potential and could be a great asset to our society. He should be given the chance.

INTRODUCTION

INTRODUCTION

"Can we learn to understand him?"
"Is there a book?"

How often these urgent words have followed my initial attempts to explain to troubled parents the nature of their child's disorder. In a desperate search for some explanation, the parents of schizophrenic children have often already consumed every book in the local library which is even remotely related to childhood emotional disturbances. A number of books are readily available which describe children who resemble the schizophrenic child, but the parents of such a child will come away from the books which describe children who are variously labeled as "emotionally disturbed", "autistic", "learning disabled with secondary emotional distress", etc. feeling as lonely and perplexed as ever.

When schizophrenia begins in childhood (accurate estimates of prevalence cannot at present be provided) its effect upon normal development is devastating. Islands of normal or even gifted functioning remain in a child who otherwise appears functionally retarded. The paradoxes in development which are seen perplex both parents and teachers, leaving all confused as to the best way of helping this child develop his potential. Too often the behavioural and sleep disturbances which accompany the disease "burn out" the family and the community school resulting in the child being institutionalized in a State or Provincial facility for the mentally ill or for the mentally retarded.

9

If this institutionalization of schizophrenic children is to be stopped teams of health and education professionals will have to become involved in planning for and managing the long term treatment of such children within the community. All the suggestions for therapeutic intervention offered in this book are dependent for their implementation upon the presence within the community of empathic and knowledgeable health professionals, as well as a committed and flexible school system. Few communities indeed are so blessed.

It is hoped that the parents of the schizophrenic child will find in this book answers to some of their questions. They will also find confirmation of some of their fears. Suggestions for positive intervention within the home itself have intentionally been kept to a minimum, as the majority of the child's disturbances in functioning, such problems as poor peer relations, impaired motor and intellectual functioning, etc. require professional intervention and peer group interaction. Ideally, the home should be maintained as a haven for this child (as it is for all normal children), a place where the child can relax and consolidate the gains which have been made in an appropriate educational and treatment facility outside the home, bizarre behaviour being disallowed in the home as soon as it is under control in the treatment facility.

It is not my intention to convey any degree of certainty regarding the long term efficacy of the suggestions for therapeutic intervention presented here. So much remains to be learned from working with schizophrenic children, from watching them grow, and from helping them develop. This book in no way pretends to be the final word.

In the hope that it will facilitate the establishment of

community-based services for schizophrenic children and their families, and in the hope that those who work with these children will find the information provided within these pages useful as a foundation upon which to build their own ability to intervene in the psychotic process, this book is now begun. A definitive solution for childhood schizophrenia must one day come forth from a biochemistry laboratory. Until then, parents, psychotherapists, teachers, and occupational therapists working together can do much to improve the functioning ability of even the most severely disabled of schizophrenic children.

Some Definitions of Terms

The term "psychotic" is used to describe persons who are moderately to severely deviant in thought, language, behaviour, and social adaptation. Two forms of psychosis occur in childhood, *childhood schizophrenia* and *infantile autism.* These two syndromes have many symptoms in common, and have—too often—been confused by both parents and professionals.

What is Schizophrenia?

The term "schizophrenia" was first used early in the 20th century by a German psychiatrist named Eugen Bleuler. This Greek word, meaning "split mind" was chosen to describe a group of patients whose emotions and thoughts were often incongruent, e.g. laughter while describing a tragic event or smiling while verbalizing hostility. Bleuler [2,3] described four cardinal symptoms in schizophrenic individuals: (1) *autism:* a preoccupation with inner stimuli (2) *ambivalence:* constantly conflicting emotions and ideas ("I love you, I hate you", "I believe in this, I also believe in that"); (3) loose *associations:* a constant switching from one subject to another which may be only remotely related; (4) a disturbance of *affect:* emotions (affects) which are either blunted (flat) or inappropriate to the context of the situation. These four symptoms have become known in psychiatry as the "four A's". They are often referred to as the *primary* symptoms of schizophrenia.

Symptoms such as delusions and hallucinations came to be emphasized in later descriptions of the illness.[4] They are often only present early in the illness or during acute exacerbations and are referred to as the *secondary* symptoms of schizophrenia.

Schizophrenia in Children

Schizophrenia in children has been the subject of much professional confusion. By now the reader may be able to guess the source of at least part of the confusion: Leo Kanner[5] took one of Bleuler's "four A's", "autism", applied it to infants, and a new disease concept was born. Controversy has raged ever since regarding the relationship of childhood-onset psychosis to adult forms of schizophrenia.[6,7] This book describes only children with symptoms *identical to* those seen in adult schizophrenia. Current usage mandates that children such as these should be diagnosed as schizophrenic.[8] In rare cases, the schizophrenic child does resemble the "autistic" child during the first few years of life.* However, by three or four years of age the behaviour of the schizophrenic child is more complex than is the behaviour of the child currently defined as "autistic" (see *autism* in "glossary of terms").

*It is probable that a great many of the children who have in the past been considered to be "high" and "middle"[9] functioning autistics would now be termed schizophrenic because they have blunted or inappropriate affect in the presence of a loosening of associations.[8] In the past children such as these were often rediagnosed as schizophrenic when they were institutionalized as adults.

The relationship—if any—between these two syndromes as presently defined remains obscure.

The diagnosis of schizophrenia at any age relies upon observing disordered thought and emotion. A positive diagnosis of childhood schizophrenia can therefore only be made when language allows the presence of either abnormal thought content (delusions or hallucinations) or abnormal thought process (fragmentation of incoming information and a loosening of association) to be documented. As a result of delayed and impoverished language development, a diagnosis in childhood can rarely be made before the fourth or fifth year of life. Since many symptoms associated with schizophrenia in children can nevertheless be easily observed in a preverbal child, the term "preschizophrenic"* has been coined for the symptomatic but preverbal infant and toddler.

Males are far more likely to develop schizophrenia before puberty than females. The reasons for this are still not known. Because of this special vulnerability, masculine pronouns have been employed throughout this book in descriptions of the schizophrenic child. When schizophrenia does begin in a female during childhood, it is likely to be first observed during the elementary school years. It is therefore often mistaken at its inception for mild mental retardation. Only rarely are symptoms noted in a female during the preschool years.

---

*The use of the term "preschizophrenic" in no way implies that the early signs of schizophrenia are unique to that disorder. Thus, for example, poor eye contact and an apparent preference for being left alone are seen in preschizophrenic, autistic, depressed and deprived infants; hypotonia is seen in preschizophrenic, mentally retarded and cerebral palsy infants; perseveration is seen in all psychotic and many brain damaged infants, etc.

An intensive investigation of schizophrenic children in this medical centre has established that at least in childhood-onset schizophrenia the motor system is significantly impaired.[10] Detailed descriptions of the motor deficits of preschizophrenic and schizophrenic children have therefore been provided throughout the text.

TO THE PARENTS

CHAPTER ONE

THE PRESCHIZOPHRENIC INFANT*
The First Three Months

The preschizophrenic infant can be most appealing. This fine-skinned infant, with the huge pupils and the wide-spaced eyes is often strikingly beautiful and appears perfectly normal. For the parents the newborn period is usually the "honeymoon".

Colic can occur as readily in preschizophrenic as in normal infants. When it does it is no different from the colic suffered by normal infants, its special significance being only that it robs the parents of any type of "honeymoon".

The Symptomatic Infant

The few infants who have symptoms of the disorder at birth are usually lethargic, "floppy" infants who sleep a great deal and feed poorly. Rarely, such an infant may even "fail to thrive" (fail to grow and gain weight) and be hospitalized. The cause of this failure to thrive is a weak suck due to poor muscle tone. This prevents the infant from getting enough calories before falling back asleep. One such four week old infant was described by the nursing staff of a children's hospital as needing three

*The descriptions of the behaviour of the preschizophrenic infant and toddler have been drawn from data volunteered to the author by the parents of schizophrenic children. Information gleaned from 22 "parent questionnaires" as well as anecdotal material from over 40 cases has been used.

hours to obtain the required three ounces of formula. (Despite this documented observation the baby left hospital with a discharge diagnosis of "inadequate mothering".)

Even the less hypotonic (poor muscle tone) preschizophrenic infant who manages to get enough nourishment to develop normally is a *slow* eater, as the lack of muscle tone interferes with both sucking and swallowing. The baby's slowness first irritates then induces guilt and feelings of inadequacy in the nourisher. Unfortunately the troubled parent who seeks any type of advice regarding these tense feeding sessions is likely to be considered "insensitive" or "impatient". Professionals and 'lay people' alike in our society have been taught to equate successful nourishing with good mothering.

About Hypotonia

Poor muscle tone in the newborn period can be associated with such deformities as "clubbed" foot, dislocated hips, or strabismus (crossed eyes). To make matters worse deformities are difficult to correct in a child whose muscle tone is poor. Even a special splint designed to correct misaligned bones may yield disappointing results.

In addition, hypotonia prevents "molding", that most endearing habit of the newborn babe (this is the medical term for the way in which newborn babies reflexly snuggle into the neck and shoulders of those who hold them). A hypotonic baby may hang limply while being lifted, or worse still may "stiffen"* each time an attempt is made to hold and cuddle. The caring parent feels

---

*No explanation can be offered at this time for the baby's "stiffening". Perhaps it represents an attempt by the "floppy" baby to voluntarily resist the pull of gravity.

somehow responsible for such behaviour, silently blaming themselves for not knowing how to "handle" this infant.

The Fearful Newborn
Not all preschizophrenic newborns are quiet, attractive babies. A few are fearful and irritable almost from the beginning. Some cannot bear being touched or held and will allow only *one* person to do so, screaming lustily when anyone else attempts to hold them. This is most unlike the normal newborn who readily learns to anticipate comfort and care from *a number of sources* (e.g. *both* parents, siblings, grandparents, etc.). The parent who is thus selected as the *only* nurturer often responds with a degree of "over-protectiveness" exposing themselves to charges of "spoiling" this babe by other family members. The baby's selection of one individual has happened so quickly that even the parent who has been thus selected may be unaware of how the situation developed. This babe has in fact begun the process of "burning out" the selected parent. Initially flattered by the baby's preference, this "chosen" parent is under tremendous strain, both because of the baby's constant demands and because of the silent resentment of other family members.

It is these fearful babies who usually manifest sleep disturbance almost from the beginning. Such babies sleep far less than the average newborn. This may be attributed by physicians and family members to precocious "alertness" and viewed as a harbinger of exceptional achievements to come.

The First Extraordinary Sense
Remarkable visual attentiveness, which inspires fantasies of special sensitivity and intelligence in the adoring parent, is common to both the unusually quiet

and the highly fearful preschizophrenic baby. By four weeks of age, this baby may be staring at a crib mobile for as long as twenty minutes [11] (in contrast to the normal one-monther whose attention span is less than five minutes). However, the parent who attempts to distract the baby from the crib mobile to his or her own face will experience the first feelings of uneasiness (again this is in contrast to normal infants who prefer the human face to an inanimate object).

Three Months to One Year

Perseveration

The most striking and alarming symptom of the preschizophrenic infant is "perseveration", or the tendency to "stick to" an activity once begun. Even awake, those infants who are symptomatic (it must be stressed that for many who will develop childhood schizophrenia there are *no* symptoms during the first year of life) can be left for long periods of time and will make no demands. As long as an object is at hand which absorbs their attention, the child will not protest. Parental ambivalence and anxiety about the ease with which this child becomes "absorbed in a world of his own" may inspire them to describe, somewhat vaguely, the baby's activities to a friend, without however inviting the friend's direct observation. A parent is then likely to be told "Stop worrying . . . and enjoy! You've got an easy baby!"

However, the distress of even the most placid of preschizophrenic infants can be as persistant as the calm. When such an infant does become upset the crying can go on for many hours (another example of perseveration). The family soon learns to avoid such upsets. Common "triggers" are identified and avoided: strangers (one infant would not allow anyone but his mother to touch him during the first year of life); loud noises (father may learn *not* to run his power tools and mother may learn to *silence* her vacuum cleaner); blankets or clothes with rough textures (this one may take a long time for parents to figure out); insects, etc.

Early Signs of Withdrawal

Both the fearful and the lethargic preschizophrenic babies begin now to select out of the environment the few objects which will preoccupy them during the next three to four years. This limited selection is in sharp contrast to the normal infant who focuses poorly, is easily distractible, and becomes excited over a wide range of stimuli. In fact, both the highly fearful and the lethargic preschizophrenic babies now begin to lose developmental ground as a result of selecting for attention and then "sticking to" only a few objects from the external environment. The difficulties of the lethargic baby are compounded by the fact that the baby is slow to reach. Only objects which come readily to hand are likely to be selected for intensive attention, thus limiting still further this baby's development.

The Pediatrician

At this stage of the preschizophrenic infant's development the family's pediatrician or family doctor if consulted, is likely to assume the role of "reassurer". Trained to observe only very gross developmental abnormalities, even the most well meaning of physicians may find little cause for concern upon examining this child. The baby after all usually sits on time and holds his head on time and rolls over on time. The doctor is likely to tell the parents to relax and enjoy this quiet baby. He may even make a small note in the child's chart: "anxious mother".

Sleep disturbance is of course a *symptom* to which a physician will respond. If the child truly sleeps only five to six hours a night, and a pattern of wakefulness has been established the physician is likely to intervene with a mild sedative. To the best of present knowledge, *chloral hydrate* (which is often prescribed) is unlikely to harm the preschizophrenic infant in any way. Attention should be paid to the stress which the child's failure to sleep causes within the family. A mild sedative is very much in order. Unfortunately, schizophrenic children often are very drug resistant. It may require very high doses of sedatives before any effect can be obtained. As a result the doctor's efforts to sedate the baby may by frustrated, although a medication such as *diphenhydramine* (benadryl) is likely to be more effective than *chloral hydrate*.

Feeding

As the child matures the slowness of his feeding may begin to be confused with "pickiness". Some of these infants are indeed also "picky". Textures appear to trouble many preschizophrenic infants. They may offer unusual resistance to tasting new foods and to switching from pureed to solid foods. Yet it is likely that the parents' best chance at introducing solid foods is during the first year of life. As the child grows older it becomes ever more difficult to introduce anything new.

The Second Year of Life

Growing Alarm

Now, this "unusual" child begins to be noticed by friends, relatives and neighbours. An intense preoccupied toddler who selectively attends to people and toys and who spends a good deal of time in simple repetitive actions troubles most observers. Close friends and relatives who initially volunteered freely to help care for this "easy" child now share parental feelings of uneasiness. The baby who had been fearful may now smile "too easily", going with anyone and everyone and using anyone and everyone to satisfy his basic needs (again this is in sharp contrast to the normal one year old, who has grown more cautious with maturation, will not smile at just anyone and will not allow just anyone to feed him and clothe him).

The preschizophrenic toddler is a puzzlement. Too little about this child's behaviour can be described in simple terms. When attempts are made to engage this child in a specific play activity, his attention span seems very short. When the child himself selects a favourite toy or occupation he can persist at it for hours. The child appears becalmed and unemotional, yet when aroused can scream or cry for several hours. The child may respond to playful teasing with a perplexed look and without a smile, yet will sit quietly by himself giggling at some unknown joke. Unable to really comprehend this child, the family may become preoccupied with his very presence in the household.

Special efforts are likely to be made to avoid upsetting the child. Almost reflexively a rigid family routine may develop. The daily bath, mealtime, bedtime, all may come to be performed in a constant and unaltered sequence. The lack of spontaneity of the preschizophrenic child may thus become the characteristic of the child's household. Unfortunately, some psychoanalysts have attached a great deal of importance to the fact that the family was rigid and controlling. Too little attention was paid to the fact that other siblings somehow managed to survive this "rigidity" without severe emotional problems!

Hypotonia Again

The majority of children who will develop the symptoms of schizophrenia before the age of three or four do not seem to have any motor impairment until the second year of life. Pictures of preschizophrenic toddlers suggest that it is some time between 16 and 24 months that the toddler who previously had manifested normal muscle tone begins to avoid sitting unsupported probably due to weak abdominal and back muscles. The child compensates unobtrusively, finding ways to sit so that he has successfully broadened his base. The favoured position is the "W" (see illustration) or with legs outstretched. Either position increases the child's base of support.

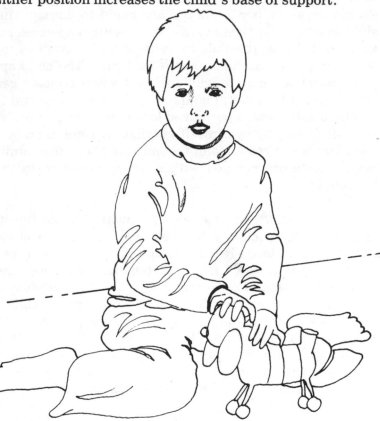

The most severely impaired preschizophrenic children tend to be late in walking. These children are also likely to drool excessively (they do not swallow very often), be very slow eaters, and resist foods which are difficult to chew. Not infrequently they have strabismus (crossed eyes) which is severe enough to require either patching or surgery. They are also prone to inguinal hernias. Since their hips rotate readily, a specialist in pediatric orthopedics may also be consulted relatively early. It would be most desirable if parents could involve physiotherapists or occupational therapists at this early stage of the child's motor development. Unfortunately, many pediatricians and family doctors tend to ignore early hypotonia in the hope that it is the syndrome called "benign congenital hypotonia". Despite the growing controversy regarding the authenticity of this syndrome many physicians continue to ignore early hypotonia in the hope that it will just "go away".

The Aimless Wanderer

The ambulatory preschizophrenic toddler wanders. This child is curious and will explore. Now the ways in which perseveration will interfere with learning can be easily observed. The normally curious toddler shifts his attention quickly from one object to another. The preschizophrenic child fixes on one particular object. Thus, the preschizophrenic toddler may begin to take pots out of the cupboards, discover the lids, and then spend the next hour putting the lids on and off the pots in a very mechanical way. The learning process is thus slowed dramatically. In a similar way the television set may be turned on and off, or its volume tuned louder and softer. To keep this child developing intellectually, the parents will have to intervene and increase the scope of the child's learning by increasing the number of objects to which the child attends. The child may actively resist any such attempt to expand his horizons.

Most distressing of all is the *nocturnal* wanderer. By the second year of life almost all preschizophrenic children have a sleep disturbance. The child may still be awake at midnight, and wake again after only four to five hours of sleep. Once awake the child will roam the house, sometimes giggling and talking to himself, more often continuing daytime explorations, which can of course injure an unsupervised toddler (such as reaching for an electric mix-master, turning on water taps, etc.). More fortunate families discover that the child will sleep when sharing a bed. Such a child may climb into bed with a sibling and fall back asleep. Pets can also be reassuring to such toddlers and the nighttime wanderer may settle on the obliging family dog.

Feeding
In extreme cases the preschizophrenic toddler may refuse any solid food whatsoever. More often, this child selects out the foods which he or she will eat and eats aggravatingly slowly. Few families will tolerate this seeming "pickiness". In the absence of professional help, the battle over food increases the tension which is already steadily developing between this parent and this child.

Early Phobias
The terror of the preschizophrenic toddler is in marked contrast to this same child's prevailing calm. Perhaps because of this contrast the family is very much shaken by the child's fears. A preschizophrenic toddler who is taken into a shopping centre may shriek and refuse to be comforted. One parent may then be delegated to sit with the child in a waiting car while the other attends to

the shopping. Similarly, this child's fear of insects may restrict the family's outings. Given the child's persistence, it requires so much energy to reassure the child that most families slip easily into a pattern of planning around the child's anxieties and fears.

Speech
During the second year of life the "language" of preschizophrenic children varies from total silence to normal language development, i.e. naming of objects and two to three word phrases. However, it is a rare schizophrenic child who develops language normally. By the end of the second year of life by far the majority of preschizophrenic children have just begun to babble. A few can also name objects. Most are very good at communicating their needs by means of pulling and gesturing (unlike autistic children).

Bonding
The bond between the preschizophrenic child and his parents is severely stressed during the second year of life. Viewing the child's seeming contentment with being alone for long periods of time, the parent often concludes that the child is "independent" and prefers to be left alone. In a very few cases this is indeed the case. However, since these toddlers are only slowly investigating the environment and learning about the world, and are selective observers of events and people, they do not need to constantly return to the parent with questions and observations. Furthermore, their fearfulness makes them cautious toddlers who risk little in movement and seldom hurt themselves. Their fascination with moving objects means that a crib mobile can prepare them for sleep as easily as a soothing parent (in fact more easily since it takes a long time for the child to settle). It requires a super parent indeed (and a most anxious one) to intrude

upon this "serene" world of the preschizophrenic toddler and not allow the child to establish himself early as a "loner".

A sickly preschizophrenic toddler or one with congenital abnormalities may demand more parental involvement, thus forging a stronger bond with the parent. Ironically therefore it is the healthy preschizophrenic child with a normal birth history and no congenital anomalies who is in the greatest danger of rupturing the parent-child bond during the first two years of life and thus establishing himself as a lonely, isolated individual.

CHAPTER TWO

THE PRESCHOOL YEARS

By two years of age there are signs of the disorder in most children in whom schizophrenia will be diagnosed before age six. In the most severely affected, lethargy, poor eye contact, constant preoccupation with a limited number of objects, and a very limited and repetitive repertoire of behaviours are the most noticeable signs. In the less severely affected a special intensity of mood, a constant excitement is the outstanding characteristic.

The Symptoms Appear

The Unpredictable

Seeming contradictions continue to be the rule in the behaviour of the preschizophrenic child. Several hours of listlessness and limited activity may be followed by an hour or two of frenetic over-activity. Perhaps as worrying as the behaviour itself is the impossibility of predicting when periods of under- and over-activity will occur. The "trigger" appears to be a perception, or a thought, or a feeling *within* the child rather than any external stimulus or anything in the child's routine (for example they are unlikely to occur "every morning" or "every evening").

The parents now become apprehensive about taking the child anywhere for fear there will be "an incident".

Still, the parents can be persuaded by friends or relatives to join in a social event. If all goes well, the parents will feel foolish for being apprehensive and may relax for awhile. There may follow a series of social outings during which all will go well and the parents will relax more and more. Before long, however, the child will embarrass the family in a social situation (e.g. a prolonged tantrum, an episode of terror, etc.) and the whole cycle of social withdrawal will resume once more.

The Disturbance in Affect

Neither the preschizophrenic nor the schizophrenic child has any ability to regulate intense emotion. The ease with which emotions explode into some form of motor activity results in the child being quickly identified as ''emotionally disturbed''. Some difficulty regulating strong emotions is normal in a child of two or three; the perseveration of the preschizophrenic child makes of this immaturity a special problem. Thus, a normal child may have a 15 to 20 minute temper tantrum; a preschizophrenic child can continue this outburst for two to three hours. Parents have reported preschizophrenic children screaming away entire nights if the parent attempted to interfere with inappropriate behaviour (a mother of a preschizophrenic child removed the calculator the child insisted upon taking to his bed and replaced it with a stuffed animal. The child screamed the entire night).

Sibling rivalry frequently becomes a major emotional trauma for both the preschizophrenic child and his family. It is not unusual for these children to attack younger siblings. When this occurs it does more to endanger the preschizophrenic child's status within the family than perhaps any other behaviour. It is important that the parents of the preschizophrenic child understand that this only represents another example of the child's tendency to *act* upon all strong emotions (in this case, jealousy). It is not an indication that the child is innately evil or sadistic.

Mannerisms

In preschizophrenic two year olds, mannerisms are common. Hand flapping which exactly resembles that seen in autism may be present. More commonly, these children show blowing, clicking, snorting, jumping up and down on one spot, rocking, head banging, or pacing back and forth. Very rarely (the author knows of only one case out of more than 40 children), the preschizophrenic child will scratch or bite himself. Usually this occurs only during temper tantrums and in no way resembles self-stimulating behaviour. In fact, most of the schizophrenic child's mannerisms (with the exception of rocking and some head banging) are in response to intense emotion. When the child becomes angry or very excited or highly anxious the mannerisms are seen. They seem to represent still another example of the ease with which strong emotions gain access to the motor system.

Poor Judgment

Normal children must be corrected several times before they will internalize a given prohibition (for example "don't run in front of cars"). The schizophrenic child may require months or even years before the successful internalization of a command occurs, perhaps because an abstract command has no impact until the child has had an experience which makes it real. An appreciation of dangerous or potentially hurtful activities is therefore slow to come. This slowness is somewhat balanced by the child's motor caution and terrified reaction to even minor injury. Nevertheless if injury is to be avoided, this child demands extra vigilance for longer periods of time from the already stressed and exhausted parent.

Hypersensitivity

The special alertness of the visual sense which the preschizophrenic child had in infancy is matched during the preschool years by the senses of hearing, smell, touch and taste. Both the immature preschizophrenic child and the more mature schizophrenic child are unable to screen out irrelevant sensory stimuli. Every sound, smell and sight strikes this child with equal intensity. Distant noises may be heeded as readily by this child as the voice of the person beside them. The child may avoid touch and protest all but the softest of clothing materials. Objects are frequently smelled before they are manipulated. All but the blandest of foods may be avoided. Objects may continue to be "mouthed" well into the fourth and fifth years of life. The sensory system of the schizophrenic child is "on" all the time, even when the child appears to be completely withdrawn. This no doubt contributes to the child's fearfulness, irritability and easy distractibility.

Disturbed Peer Relations and Play Behaviour

Throughout the preschool years the schizophrenic child prefers the company of adults to that of his peers. When in the company of his peers, this child will play *beside* them until well past the age when most normal children have begun interactive play. The schizophrenic child prefers building toys, puzzles, and toy vehicles to aggressive toys such as guns, or toys which inspire projective play (fantasy play) such as dolls and houses. Often this child is fearful of toys, suspecting that anything which looks that real *is* real and should be handled with great caution. Not infrequently the child prefers numbers, letters, and noiseless machines such as calculators to toys of any kind. Many of these children must be actively involved in play by a knowledgeable adult. Otherwise they will sit for long hours passively observing television (often preferring the commercials to the actual shows; or perseverating in a number or a letter activity.

Hypotonia Again

The complex motor activities which must be mastered during the preschool years present great difficulty to the hypotonic schizophrenic child. Activities such as walking downstairs, throwing a ball, catching a ball, turning faucets on and off, and riding a bicycle will require some help from knowledgeable adults before any degree of mastery can be achieved. A few of these children are toe walkers. Almost all of these children broaden their base (feet wide apart) and hold their arms well away from their sides while they walk.

Anxiety Begins

Difficulty falling asleep, frequent wakefulness at night, and unusual fearfulness, all of which are usually first encountered in the preschizophrenic child during the second year of life are encountered in almost all schizophrenic children by the third and fourth year of life. The child's vulnerability to phobias now complicates the toilet training process. Many a schizophrenic child has found the roar of the flushing toilet an unpleasant enough experience to warrant avoidance behaviour. Once the child becomes anxious or oppositional, toilet training may prove very nearly impossible to accomplish during the preschool years.

Language Development

The acquisition of language is the major developmental milestone achieved by all normal children by the end of the third year of life. Not so the schizophrenic child. More than seventy-five percent of schizophrenic children are language delayed. Even the few preschizophrenic children who had been able to name objects and use two to three word phrases during the second year of life, often appear to lose this ability during the third year of life (it is difficult to know for certain whether the child has truly lost the ability to talk, is too anxious to talk, is too oppositional to talk, or is too lethargic to talk).

At the beginning of the fourth year of life the majority of preschizophrenic children are brought to a child development facility as a result of "speech delay". Usually the child then possesses a great deal of unintelligible speech. A number of behaviours are also evident which communicate to the child's caretaker exactly what the child wants. As a rule this child uses gestures and makes good eye contact when he is communicating basic needs and he appears to comprehend most of what is said to him. Despite severe language problems, these children are therefore not usually very frustrated by their early attempts at communication.

The most common history of language development for schizophrenic children is a prolonged period of babbling, followed by a period of unintelligible speech, followed by a period during which more than half of the language is echoing and delayed echoing (such as the repetition of commercials and nursery rhymes), until finally the child develops somewhat sparse and agrammatic speech in which connecting words are often omitted and loosely associated themes are featured. The schizophrenic child seldom uses the pronouns "I" and "you", preferring to use proper names. Neologisms ("new words") are a part of the speech of more than half of schizophrenic children. Many schizophrenic children are fascinated by the sound of certain words. These children may use a word for no other reason than because they like repeating it, and they may combine words because they

like the way they sound together ("clang associations"*).
Some parents become expert translators.**

Consultations Begin

Most often it is between the fourth and sixth year of
life that the schizophrenic child begins to be evaluated by
various health professionals. Presenting complaints are
most often "speech delay", "preoccupation with his own
world", hyperactivity, negativisim, temper tantrums,
isolation from peers, etc. Each discipline that sees the
child tends to describe the deficit relevant to that discipline. Thus, speech therapists may view the child as an
"expressive aphasia". Neurologists and child development specialists view the child as "developmentally
delayed", "mildly retarded", "perceptually handicapped", "on the autistic continuum", or "atypical autistic". Educators view the child as potentially "learning
disabled" (it should be immediately emphasized that
although many schizophrenic children are initially labelled as "learning disabled" the converse is *not* true, the
vast majority of learning disabled children are *not* schizophrenic). There exist "experts" who will view the child as
primarily motorically disabled. Child psychiatrists view
the child as a "childhood psychosis".* For the parent the
long hunt for an answer has begun.

*In response to the therapist saying "That's true" a four year old schizo-
phrenic replied "Meat Stew".

**A four year old stated that he had "Tires for the sun". His mother explained
he was describing his father's custom of changing the tires on the car every
spring from winter tires to regular tires.

*Lauretta Bender [12] a psychiatrist who devoted herself to the study of child-
hood schizophrenia, once described this disorder as a "*pan*disorder" (signify-
ing that the disorder involved *all* systems). Little wonder then that each discipline which examines the child will be confronted by a relevant deficit.

CHAPTER THREE

THE PRESCHOOL YEARS
IN A DAYCARE SETTING

It is difficult to predict where the preschizophrenic or schizophrenic child will encounter the first group setting. For some, who are placed in a day care centre during infancy, group living may begin in early infancy.

Infancy

The quiet, preschizophrenic babe is likely to be viewed as a "good" baby in a day care setting. Even a perceptive caretaker is unlikely to become uneasy until the child is six or seven months old. The tendency of the child to focus on but a few objects will probably go unnoticed during the first few months of life.

The irritable and fearful preschizophrenic baby will of course be a source of difficulty in a day care setting. This child may be viewed as highly troublesome, and in fact the parent may be asked to withdraw the child by two or three months of age. A group setting offers far more sensory stimulation than a quiet home setting, and it is extremely difficult to shelter an irritable baby from excessive sensory stimulation in such a group setting.

It is probable that well-trained day care staff will detect the symptomatic infant's repetitiveness and tendency to perseverate much earlier than a new and inexperienced mother. Certainly by the time the preschizophrenic infant is eight to ten months of age one would expect the day care staff to note both the hyper-sensitivity and the perseveration of the symptomatic infant. In many cases, the staff may assume that this is an unusually intelligent baby, since the intensity with which the preschizophrenic baby studies objects can indeed appear to presage special "giftedness".* Thus, the quiet babies who display sensory precocity are likely to arouse little concern in day care staff. Such staff are accustomed to receiving highly variable amounts of affection from the infants in their care. If the preschizophrenic infant appears somewhat aloof, the staff will assume that the baby relates much better to his own parents.

Ambulation and Socialization

The first true difficulties are likely to be encountered when the preschizophrenic baby begins to walk. This child is much less responsive to the group, and much more responsive to his own internal reactions. Although at times this child may imitate others in the group, at other times he may act as if there is no one else present, even walking directly over other children or knocking them heedlessly to one side. This baby will take whatever he wishes, sometimes picking up an object from in front of another or even from someone's grasp without the slight-est acknowledgement that the object is in anyone's possession.

"Emotional Disturbance"

In a group setting the "emotional disturbance" of the preschizophrenic child will be observed almost as soon as it appears. Perhaps the most disquieting symptom of all is the "mirthless" laugh (reported to have occurred in a

*Not only are most childhood schizophrenics visually alert, some are highly artistic. There have been great artists who suffered from schizophrenia.

preschizophrenic infant as young as six months), the tone-
less laugh of the preschizophrenic two year old which
seems unconnected to any observable source of humour.
Equally striking is the child's failure to respond emotionally in group situations, and in fact the child's relative
lack of emotional responsiveness to anything external. All
emotion in a child like this appears to be generated from
within.

Except in the highly irritable symptomatic child,
temper tantrums are less likely to be a problem for the
preschizophrenic toddler in a group setting than at home.
All group settings have some routine and structure to
which the child becomes accustomed. There is seldom any
disruption in that routine, especially during the infant and
toddler stage. The noise level in a group setting tends to
be more constant, rather than variable as in a home
(where quiet may alternate with such noises as power
tools and vacuum cleaners). Nap times, which are part of
the routine of the daycare nursery, are not usually prob-
lematic even for the symptomatic infant. If a child has
established a regular daily routine, the day care staff is
unlikely to interfere. In many ways a group setting is a far
less emotionally charged atmosphere than a home setting.
Thus it is that in a daycare setting temper tantrums are
unlikely to become a significant problem much before
three to four years of age for the symptomatic infant or
toddler.

Feeding

Eating activities provide a rare time when the child-
care workers have a really excellent opportunity to view
the disabilities of the symptomatic child. The poor coordination of chewing and tongue movements, the drooling,
the slowness of the eating pace, all should attract the
attention of child-care staff. If the child is an irritable,

fearful child, the staff may view the child's slow eating behaviour as still another example of oppositionalism. In a child who is withdrawn and quiet however, the slow eating will not be mistaken for resistance, but will arouse true concern. A perceptive staff may then begin to notice other aspects of the child's motor development and may express some concern to the parents. Some preschizophrenic children are initially mistaken for the mildly retarded, who also demonstrate poor muscle tone and some apathy. More frequently, the staff will be puzzled by the child's uneven performance (the poor motor tone coupled with the sensory alertness and the ease with which the child learns certain tasks) and will articulate their puzzlement to the family.

The First Strengths

During the second and third year of a child's life in a group setting the ease with which the preschizophrenic masters certain tasks also attracts attention. These children are often very quick at anything resembling puzzles and are fascinated by mechanical objects. They will usually gravitate to such toys or to stereos or tape recorders, and may outshine their peers in their ability to manipulate them. As a result, daycare personnel may discount many of their concerns regarding the child's otherwise delayed development. The staff is likely to assure themselves that in the presence of such ability, whatever difficulties there are will soon disappear.

CHAPTER FOUR

NURSERY SCHOOL
AND KINDERGARTEN

By the time most schizophrenic children enter a nursery school programme at three and a half to four years of age, many symptoms of the disease are well established. Those children who have already been examined by a professional (more than half of the children in whom a definitive diagnosis can be made during the fourth year of life) are likely to have been referred to a programme that is designed for language disabled children or will be accompanied into a regular programme by an aide who has been especially hired to allow this integration to occur. No matter which of these two alternatives* are followed the teacher of the schizophrenic child must have a good understanding of the child's problems.

Group Behaviour

One way of viewing schizophrenia is as a failure to form a sense of self. The most lucid way of conceptualizing this is as a deficit in the "ego boundary"[13] or as an impaired sense of separate existence. This deficit in the ego boundary is never more evident than in the three or four year old schizophrenic child who is placed in a group

---

*Many communities offer neither a programme for language disabled children nor an aide to stay beside the child. If parents are offered no alternative or are told to place their child in a facility for the mentally retarded they should actively resist. A visit to the nearest Child Development or Child Psychiatry clinic is recommended.

situation. The child goes where he pleases, takes what he wants, and frequently seems to be almost unaware of the other children in the room. Adults are rarely similarly ignored by the schizophrenic child. Perhaps because adults loom so large to the eyes of a child, even the schizophrenic child appears to recognize the separate power and authority of the adult figure. It is interesting to speculate that this is why the child prefers adult company (i.e. his sense of being a separate person is less threatened).

It should be stressed that as with everything else the tendency of the schizophrenic child to ignore his peers is not a consistent tendency. At times, higher functioning schizophrenic children who conceptualize in grandiose ways may attempt to incorporate the children in their immediate environment into a delusional system. This emerges as very "bossy" behaviour as the schizophrenic child will order everything in this interaction from what the other children are allowed to say to what they are allowed to do, e.g. if the child has decided that everything which resembles a wire in the room is to be designated as a wire, all the wire-like objects in the classroom will be confiscated, and every child who is holding a wire-like object will be told exactly what it represents, how to hold it and what must next be done with it. What is consistent is that the child treats all individuals as if they were extensions of himself. He cannot comprehend that they may have ideas and wishes of their own.

What has just been described is the rather limited way in which the schizophrenic child interacts with others from time to time. Most of the time, in a group setting even the highest functioning schizophrenic child will avoid all contact with his peers. This child will choose to play by himself as far away from others as is permitted, and with a rather limited number of toys. The child's preference will be for building, either by putting together puzzles or by using actual building toys such as wooden blocks or Lego. Frequently letters and numbers are also sources of fascination for a schizophrenic child, water play is enjoyed, and ''Play-Doh'' will be mouthed, smelled and kneaded rather than molded into shapes. The most outstanding characteristic of the child's play is its repetitiveness (also known as ''stereotypy''). The child ''sticks to'' (perseverates) a single activity for an astonishingly long time. Yet, all efforts to introduce a new activity to the child are confronted by a seemingly ''short attention span''. The teacher, like the parent during the child's infancy, is puzzled by this paradoxical behaviour.

Eye Contact
The three year old schizophrenic tends to avoid eye contact. In this, the child resembles the classically autistic child. However, one important difference is that the schizophrenic child always makes eye contact when identifying one of his needs. In fact, as the child matures, difficulties regulating eye contact occur more obviously as one of many signs that the child does not comprehend social norms. When this child does make eye contact it will be to stare inappropriately.

''Hyperactivity''
It seems to be between the ages of three and seven that the schizophrenic child has the highest energy level. Since the child has very little ability to regulate himself, this high energy may resemble that of the hyperactive child. The important differentiators are the child's highly *variable* attention span and the fact that the schizophrenic child's periods of ''hyperactivity'' take the form of either totally *aimless* activity (as opposed to short spurts of goal directed behaviour in the true hyperactive child) or spurts of *stereotyped* activity (such as episodes of rapid pacing or

jumping up and down on one spot). In the most severely motorically affected, motor activity is notably jerky or clumsy.

The Subtypes of Schizophrenia*

Schizophrenia in childhood presents itself in three forms. The most severely affected children (and by far the rarest) belong to the *"disorganized type"*, whose title is self-explanatory. The majority of the children belong to the *"undifferentiated type"*, i.e. they have features of several different types of schizophrenia. The most high functioning children (although the most dangerous to society) belong to the *"paranoid type"*, which is characterized by the development of delusional systems which are either persecutory or grandiose (or both) in nature.

The Paranoid Schizophrenic

It is this child who *must* be identified during the pre-elementary school years. Once this child enters the structured classroom of the elementary school years he may go undetected until junior high school when his difficulty comprehending the increasingly abstract academic material which must be mastered will become apparent. In the nursery school and kindergarten setting he can be easily identified as the child who prefers to be alone, communicates freely only with the grown-ups in the classroom, interacts with his peers only at the level described above (where he assigns them tasks and ideas) and appears strangely preoccupied and intense for one so young.

It is this child who is often a constant questioner. His anxiety level is very high and all his senses are

*The definitions of subtypes which are used here have been taken from the Diagnostics and Statistics Manual III.[8]

extraordinarily alert. His questions are perseverative, and can never be satisfied with an answer. They range from "Why is the sky blue?" to "How come the sky doesn't fall down?" to "Why can't I fly?". The teacher is often convinced that this child is unusually intelligent. His inability to accept answers or be reassured is however disquieting. In fact, his compulsive questioning can probably best be understood by comparing it with the religious preoccupation of the late adolescent paranoid schizophrenic (who often becomes preoccupied with questions relating to the purpose of life and death, the so-called "existential crisis").

The paranoid schizophrenic child has no sense of what is trivial, nor can he be taught to appreciate the difference between trivialities and relevancies. It is difficult to reassure him or answer his questions. He will remember every detail of a teacher's response to his question and will express great perplexity (and may even become enraged) if the teacher attempts to give a fuller and more comprehensive answer to a question which had previously been answered in a more simple and concrete way.

It should be stressed that it is only during these preelementary school years that this child is a verbal "questioner". By the seventh or eighth year of life this child no longer values others sufficiently to ask questions. He will then begin to construct his own answers based upon extremely faulty information. When he stops asking questions and begins inventing his own answers, true paranoia begins.

Disordered Thinking

All schizophrenic children are thought disordered. In the most low functioning schizophrenic child thought is completely "fluid", i.e. it is totally lacking in organization. In the more highly functioning schizophrenic child some organization of thought does occur, all too often along delusional lines. Very early in human development thought which is either totally lacking in organization or is organized in a very simple way should be restricted to the dream state and to the unconscious.[14] During the waking state, normal thought is tightly organized into groups of ideas or concepts. In the thought disordered schizophrenic disorganized or poorly organized thought is never totally suppressed and may even be the dominant thought process.

The Importance of Context

The normal three to four year old child has already begun to appreciate context, i.e. to acquire an awareness of "what goes with what". The schizophrenic child appears to be completely unable to note context. All incoming information is learned and apparently stored as fragments which are devoid of context. Thus, a schizophrenic child will learn that a pizza is round, that an apple pie is round, and that both are made of dough. He may then ask for an "apple pizza", but will shriek with rage if anybody offers him apples as a topping on pizza in the mistaken belief that that is what he wishes. All that has happened is that two concepts that have something in common have been mistakenly juxtaposed (a "condensation"). Similarly, because the slice of a lemon and the face of a clock resembled each other in shape, a four year old schizophrenic child wondered aloud if a lemon would "ring" (like daddy's alarm clock) or if he could "eat" the face of a clock. It would seem then that not only is information stored away within the brain in fragments, but it is subject to recall and recombination with material which may be only slightly related. The result is marked illogicality.

Illogicality and Negativism

The illogical associations of the schizophrenic child are at times not that deviant from the kind of associative errors that normal children make. In combination with the tendency of the schizophrenic child to perseverate and to be oppositional these illogical associations become a major impediment to learning. Thus, a schizophrenic child of four and a half had come to think of television antennas as "roof antennas". When an attempt was made to explain to him that they were in fact television antennas he angrily shouted "no", ran about yelling "roof antenna" and persisted in this angry outburst for ten minutes. He did finally accept that the purpose of the antenna was as stated and that people did in fact call them "television antennas" rather than "roof antennas". Once he learned this, he very quickly mastered the concept that the antennas on cars were for the radios. For the next week he went about constantly telling anyone who would listen what he had learned about television and radio antennas. The importance of this anecdote is that it not only illustrates the special learning problems of the schizophrenic child, but it also highlights how these difficulties may be overcome. These children will learn, but the pace at which they will learn is very much modified by their tendency to perseverate, fragment, ignore context, and be oppositional.

Disordered Language

It is axiomatic that a thought disorder will be reflected in disordered language. In childhood schizophrenia two extremes in communication styles are seen: Children whose speech is sparse and impoverished (poverty of speech) and children with marked pressure of speech. Each of these extremes may represent an attempt on the child's part to organize thought. Certainly, when excitement leads to an increase in disorganization, children with impoverished speech may talk a great deal (but make very little sense) and children with pressure of speech may find themselves stuttering and unable to talk.

Neologisms and Word Approximations

About fifty percent of schizophrenic children make up new words which appear to have no relationship to existing words. One such child used to write neologisms beside his drawings. The drawing provided clues as to the meaning of the neologisms (see illustration p. 48).

Word approximations are easier to understand. They very much resemble the word the child is attempting to say, for example "fairways" in place of "freeways". At three to four years of age word approximations are very much a part of the normal child's speech. They will however remain a part of the schizophrenic's speech throughout life.

Word Salad

Word salad (or a series of loosely related words*) is commonly seen in schizophrenic children between three

---

*The term *verbigeration* was used in the old psychiatry literature. Current usage includes word salad under the rubric of "Incoherence".

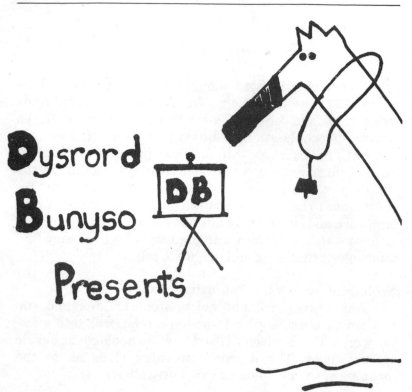

Dysrord
Bunyso DB
Presents

and six years of age. In the most severely affected more than seventy-five percent of their language may consist of words which have little or no relationship to each other: "Who's off the chair, mommy, out of the chair, Snoopy's on the chair, knee, tree, chair, cars on the chair . . .". What can be seen in this quotation which constitutes the verbalization of a six year old schizophrenic child is that the words are bound together by an element in common (the chair) or by a clang association ("knee, tree"). As these children learn new words, they tend to use them fairly frequently often appearing to be practising the word. A great deal of the child's communication may consist of these newly learned words or concepts.

Echolalia and Delayed Echolalia

Normal children also begin learning language through echoing. However, normal children seem to learn at a relatively early age to repeat words silently to themselves rather than state them aloud. Thus, by three or four years of age, it is rare to hear a normal child echo a word. The schizophrenic child however continues to echo words and even phrases throughout the developmental years. It may be that this process represents still another rupture of the "ego boundary" or the ability to contain within oneself thought or emotion.

Every individual knows the experience of having songs "echoing" in the head or remembering commercials or rhymes. The echoing *aloud* of rhymes or commercials however is not seen in normal children until much later when it constitutes a part of group interaction and play, i.e. the normal child only sings commercials when his peers are similarly engaged. The schizophrenic child may produce a television commercial—or any other relevant remembered fragment (a "delayed echo") in response to a language stimulus. Thus, one schizophrenic child overheard his therapist and teacher discussing the need for a vacation and burst out with "you deserve a break today" (the McDonald's commercial at the time).

Unintelligible Speech and Talking to Oneself

Very early in development a schizophrenic child who communicates only minimally with others may be observed to be playing by himself and talking away. If one attempts to move closer and tries to overhear what the child is saying much of the language is incomprehensible. Isolated words can be heard, but the child will often fall silent if anyone approaches. The contrast between the sparsity of the speech which the child uses when interacting with others and the seeming torrent of words which can be overheard when the child is playing alone is striking indeed. This behaviour resembles entirely that of the adult schizophrenic who can be seen in the streets talking to him or herself.

The Regulation of Voice

The schizophrenic child often speaks so softly that he can barely be heard. Yet in the next moment the same child may speak in an astonishingly loud voice. There is reason to believe that not only does the child have difficulty understanding that voice must be regulated, the child seems to lack the ability to judge when he is speaking softly and when he is speaking loudly. The loud voice of the schizophrenic child can be strikingly monotonous. It is highly irritating to the listener, and has at times been identified for the author as the single most irritating characteristic of the young schizophrenic child. The voice can perhaps best be characterized as mechanical or computer-like. The speech is very precise and formal, most likely analogous to the formalistic speech which has been described in adult schizophrenics.

Disordered Balance and Motor Function

The Gait of the Schizophrenic Child

Most young childhood schizophrenics have an abnormal gait. A few toe-walk until they are five or six years of age. This in no way reflects a tight heel cord in these children. More commonly, the gait of these children is broad-based and characterized by a Chaplinesque slapping of the foot. The arms tend to be held stiffly and slightly out from the side in a parachute-like position. There is much about this child's gait which suggests a disturbance in balance [15].

Balance

Here again we have contradictions. Early in development the schizophrenic child may dislike being tossed into the air or having his balance disrupted in any way ("anti-gravity play"). Later, the same child may relish being constantly spun around (as on a merry-go-round or ferris wheel) and may perseverate endlessly at this type of play. It is noteworthy that these children appear to depend for balance upon their eyes [16]. Such a child will not willingly play "pin the tail on the donkey", and will resist in every way any attempt to interfere with the use of his eyes. He will *not* walk backwards and he will avoid complex balance activities, such as a balance beam.

Gross and Fine Motor Functioning

There is evidence that the gross motor system is more severely affected than the fine motor system in schizophrenic children [16]. At age three or four, however, these children have difficulty with both modes of functioning. During the preschool years it is difficult for these children to learn to hold a crayon properly or to control the first attempts at eye-hand coordination. This is in fact likely to be the first evidence of "learning disability" that the teacher will note. Yet, as the child gains better control of his limbs this early dysfunction should cease to be significant. Some schizophrenic children have become extraordinary artists despite never learning to hold a pencil normally. It is therefore important that too much emphasis not be placed upon the child's eye-hand problems. The author knows of one schizophrenic child who by twelve years of age had absolutely no evidence of visual motor dysfunction, but who continued to be highly fearful of writing.

During the nursery and kindergarten years the schizophrenic child is unlikely to encounter any serious problems with group activities as a result of poor motor functioning. This is because all children lack motor skills at this age. The gap between the gross motor functioning of the schizophrenic child and the normal child will become evident only later, during the elementary school years. It is therefore important during the nursery and kindergarten years to make every effort to keep the schizophrenic child involved in group activities with normal children. Soon enough the schizophrenic child will find himself unable to compete motorically with his peers.

Strategies for Intervention

Perseveration

Perhaps the most important symptom which those who interact with the child should try to correct is that of perseveration. It is this tendency which interferes most with the child's ability to acquire new information. The child's tendency to get "stuck" in a very limited range of behaviours and ideas should be controlled as much as possible by the child-care staff or nursery and kindergarten school teachers responsible for the child's care. A very helpful way to intervene is to hire an aide who will be beside the child throughout the nursery school or kindergarten programme to insure that the child participates in the group activities. This will prevent the child from drifting out to the periphery of every circle activity and keep the child imitating group behaviour. The aide functions as an "auxiliary ego*" for the child, keeping the child on task.

---

*"Ego" is the term applied to that part of the psyche which is responsible for self-regulation. It is the task of the "ego" to insure that the individual's innermost drives and wishes are satisfied in socially acceptable ways. The term "ego" therefore describes the executive function of the mind with the power to regulate all functions including thought, affect, voice and movements.[17,18]

Inattention to Context

The nursery school or kindergarten teacher who teaches a schizophrenic child will themselves have to have a heightened awareness of context. The ability of normal children to learn concepts in context is one which is easily taken for granted. The presence of a schizophrenic child in the group will sharpen the teacher's sensitivity to this issue. Again, if an aide has been hired, the aide can take a moment to point out ("reality test") the context of whatever is being taught to the schizophrenic child.

A special warning is in order here regarding stories and films which anthropomorphize inanimate objects (e.g. a train which talks). The schizophrenic child may identify with the inanimate object and perseverate for days on himself being a train, or a vegetable, etc. The child has failed to notice that this is "pretend" and in his puzzlement and rage acts out the story. The teacher or aide must remember to point out to the child that in real life, we all know, trains do not talk!

Illogicality and Negativism

Extra time should be taken to explain to schizophrenic children that the context in which a word is found can sometimes *define* the meaning (e.g. "to", "two" and "too" are defined by context). Teachers should be sensitive to the fact that if the child drifts off or is disruptive it is often because the child has lost contact with the group. Most often, this is due to the child's failure to comprehend, or because the teacher has inadvertently upset the child by redefining something the child thought he understood (the example of the "television antenna" when the child preferred "roof antenna"). The child's negative responses to such changes should be dealt with firmly and kindly. Often it is useful to have a corner of the room where the schizophrenic child can be asked to sit quietly until he regains control of himself. The child will after awhile learn to go on his own to "sit and think" until the torrent of thoughts and emotions has settled. This technique can avoid a lot of temper tantrums.

Group Behaviour and Eye Contact

It is not wise to make a big fuss over eye contact. The child will be more responsive to an urging, "please look at me", than to an order to "look at me". The teacher should appreciate that the very weak sense of self is a source of panic to the schizophrenic child. The child's preoccupation with inner stimuli and avoidance of eye contact may help the child to preserve a sense of separateness. It is wise to respect the child's need to cultivate some sense of separation, since the alternative is a total disintegration of the personality. Rather than insisting upon eye contact on a one-to-one basis, the wise teacher will help the child to feel comfortable in the group and not isolate himself in a corner, while letting the child decide how much he wishes to look at individuals in the group.

The child's tendency to treat other children in the classroom as if they were not there must be kindly but firmly dealt with. It is very important to teach children like this concepts of ownership. This will strengthen their own sense of self and help them to understand that others have an existence apart from them. These children should not be allowed to take whatever they wish. They should be directed to notice that other children are playing with the object, and made to wait their turn. The teacher should not be swayed by the fact that the schizophrenic child readily loses interest in an object if he must wait for it. Instead, a way should be found to re-interest him in the object at a more appropriate time.

It is especially important to attempt to make contact with the paranoid schizophrenic child. This child should not be allowed to involve other children in his fantasies. Instead some effort should be made to encourage him to project his fantasies onto toys while the difference between reality and fantasy is stressed (even though it may appear to be early in development for such a difference to be emphasized).

Despite the fact that this child will resist any attempts at changing his patterns of interaction, every effort should be made to make him less idiosyncratic and to interrupt his grandiosity. (E.g. a five year old once informed the author that he weighed one million pounds, and that when he grew up he would build a telephone system *on top* of the ocean [instead of underwater]. This same child had tried to move the playroom wall because he did not like where it was.) Early psychiatric intervention is essential for this child, who above all needs to learn to share his perceptions with others and to make some sort of peace with consensual validation.

Disordered Language
The schizophrenic child (who has demonstrated repeatedly that he has achieved total language comprehension) should be encouraged gently but firmly to articulate his thoughts in sentence form. This is the intervention to correct "poverty of speech". Conversely the schizophrenic child who talks compulsively and constantly needs to be taught that not every thought that crosses his mind need be articulated. He should be helped to understand that there is such a thing as *silent* thought.

Echoing and delayed echoing should be gently discouraged. The child should be helped to find an alternative to a television commercial for expressing the idea he has just articulated. A tape recorder can be used to help the child develop a concept of voice modulation. Indeed, it is hoped that before long speech therapists will develop a series of well-recognized strategies for dealing with each of the aspects of the speech and language disorders of schizophrenic children (including the all-too-common articulation defect).

The child whose language is mostly word salad will require much patience. It should be appreciated by the teacher that this child is still mastering the *naming* of objects. The child will need time to gain some confidence before too much emphasis is placed upon sentences.

Finally, the schizophrenic child should not be allowed to talk aloud to himself in a public place. This should be kindly but firmly stopped. This is part of instructing the child to notice the presence of others. Forcing him to keep his fantasies to himself will also strengthen his sense of self.

The Role of Play Therapy

The normal child projects much of the real world onto toys and achieves a sense of mastery by playing with and manipulating these imitations of reality [19] . Many schizophrenic children are too fearful of the close resemblance of play objects to reality to engage in projective play. Play therapy can be very helpful to such children if the therapist is comfortable with the role of interpreting reality (''this is pretend'') to a child whose reality testing (ability to separate fantasy from reality) is significantly impaired. If good therapeutic gains are to be made the therapist will have to be sensitive to all the issues *re* disordered thinking and to respect the child's need for separation. (Since psychosexual conflicts only rarely surface in the play material of a three to five year old schizophrenic child, they will be discussed in the next chapter.)

Disordered Balance and Motor System

It is highly desirable that schizophrenic children participate in a gross motor therapy programme as soon as possible. If none of the child's teachers have any expertise in this area appropriate consultations should be arranged. A qualified occupational therapist can devise a programme for a motorically impaired child which can be implemented in the nursery school or kindergarten. By the time the child reaches elementary school his impaired motor functioning will interfere greatly with interpersonal relations. Early interventions are therefore essential.

Hypotonia coupled with loose joints provides very little bodily resistance to movement. The resulting decrease in "feedback" to the central nervous system almost certainly interferes with the development of the ability to control and modify movement and may contribute to the persistence in many schizophrenic children of some aspects of the sensorimotor stage of cognitive development (during which the toddler learns by engaging in repetitive motor activities, such as rolling objects back and forth [20]). The child's body concept and therefore his sense of self may be improved by means of devices which increase the amount of feedback the child receives while moving (e.g. small weights attached to the child's arms, having the child move in mediums such as sand or water, etc.).

"Mainstreaming"*

When first identified the preschool schizophrenic

---

*Mainstreaming for some represents an educational ideology which insists that *all* handicapped children must be educated with non-handicapped children. The author believes that an individual educational plan must be made for each disturbed child.

child benefits most from at least a year in a highly specialized setting wherein much emphasis is placed upon
controlling psychotic behaviours (motor mannerisms,
total isolation, etc.). Following this, the child who is *no
more than a year behind developmentally*, can begin the
process of integration in a group setting with normal
peers, initially on a part-time basis. It should be continued
only as long as no significant regression occurs.

The kindergarten year, with its relatively non-
competitive programme, provides an excellent opportunity to integrate high-functioning schizophrenic children with their normal peers. The schizophrenic child may
realize many advantages from being thus placed. Motor
mannerisms (blowing, clicking, etc.), with firm intervention, can be kept to a minimum. If the group is small, it is
not too difficult to persuade the high-functioning schizophrenic child to join.

The size of the group is critical. The inability of the
schizophrenic child to screen out extraneous sensory
stimuli makes a too-stimulating environment a nightmare
for this child. Some efforts will have to be made to insure
that even the highest functioning schizophrenic child is
placed in a group of no more than twenty during these
pre-school years. Even a group of that size (which in the
regular kindergarten programme is likely to break into
three or four smaller groups for the purpose of most activities) can present major difficulties to the paranoid
schizophrenic child (whose senses appear to be the most
alert of all). It will require much tact and sensitivity from
the supervising adult to persuade this child to move towards the group (getting him within two feet of group
activity can be viewed as a major achievement!). As it is
crucial to decrease this child's social isolation, if he persists in remaining aloof a small special needs programme

in which he feels safe enough to participate is preferable to integration into a normal kindergarten programme.

The "undifferentiated" type of the schizophrenic child (who has some disorganization and some paranoia), who is high-functioning will probably have one of his best growing up years in the sixth year of life. This child's expressive language at about five should be less than one year behind if he has already received a few years of good and intensive care. With some attention to all the difficulties which have already been described he will feel fairly safe at this age and will not find it too difficult to compete with normal children (many of whom will not be much further ahead than he is).

Neither normal children nor schizophrenic children are motorically very sophisticated during the kindergarten year. Although the schizophrenic child is usually a year or more behind in motor development he will be able to join normal children in most climbing and swinging activities (provided a sensitive teacher gives considerable emotional support to the fearful schizophrenic child). Running will usually present little difficulty, since normal children do not run very quickly at this age and young children tend to be quite tolerant of each other's awkwardness. Competing motorically with normal peers may actually benefit the schizophrenic child provided the child can avoid feeling overwhelmed and can experience some success.

The only schizophrenic child who will be unable to derive benefit from exposure to a regular kindergarten programme during the preschool years is the "disorganized type". This child, even with the help of an aide, will be too disruptive to be included in the larger group setting. This child will require a group of no more than six to eight children. If a small group could be provided, it would be desirable for even this child to be exposed to normal peers during the preschool years since such exposure would help to keep motor mannerisms and bizarre behaviour to a minimum. The difficulty with placing this child in a large group is that with any kind of stimulation this child will swing into disruptive behaviour. He will not sit still, he will wander constantly about the room and he will continue the behaviour described earlier of walking over people and ignoring their presence. He will frequently be agitated, excited, irritable, and manifest constant emotional overflow. There may be noise mannerisms (wailing while moving, repetitive loud noises coupled to movements, etc.) and episodes of uncontrollable laughing and crying. With firm controls, and efforts to keep sensory stimulation within limits, this child can settle. Usually, preschool programmes for children such as this will have to be hospital-based in order to ensure that paramedical personnel such as occupational therapists and psychiatric nurses are included in the treatment team.

The most undesirable placement for schizophrenic children is with children suffering from *primary* mental retardation. Such placement will be followed by either a marked increase in motor mannerisms, emotional excitement and disruptive behaviour, or an increase in social withdrawal and preoccupation with internal stimuli. Most schizophrenic children are quite capable of mastering a standard academic curriculum once their disordered way of thinking is appreciated and suitable strategies are devised by the teacher. The restricting factor will be the *rate* at which the child learns, rather than *how much* the child learns. (Some of these children will learn only when steps have been taken to shut out sensory stimuli, such as when they are placed in an enclosed space with earphones in place and they are obliged to receive all of their learning from *one* visual and *one* auditory source, a technique made possible by the development of such systematized ways of learning as the computer-based *System 80*). If schizophrenic children are placed with retarded children they will receive much too little cognitive stimulation. Secondary mental retardation is the inevitable consequence of such placement.

CHAPTER FIVE

ELEMENTARY SCHOOL

Very few schizophrenic children will be able to enter a regular grade I programme. Most will require a special needs programme where treatment approaches are emphasized. Even schizophrenic children with intellectual functioning well within the normal range, who could handle a full academic programme, will find competing with normal children in a regular-sized classroom extremely stressful. Stress which exceeds the child's capacity to cope will result in an increase in psychotic symptoms and a severe inhibition of cognitive development, i.e. the child will stop learning.

Some high-functioning schizophrenic children will be able to "keep up" in a regular classroom well into the elementary school years. However, integration with normal children appears to be helpful to the schizophrenic child only as long as the child remains unaware of his own deficits in functioning. Unfortunately, the more intelligent and aware the schizophrenic child is, the keener is this child's awareness of his own deficits in functioning. As soon as "scapegoating" by normal peers begins, or the schizophrenic child shows signs of withdrawal and increasing social isolation, or there is an increase in psychotic symptomatology, alternative ways of educating the schizophrenic child should be sought. In particular, an increase in paranoid ideation ("when I grow up I'm going to live on a desert island all by myself'') or delusional ideation (one seven year old who had not allowed anyone to touch *him* for several years began to react to observing *others* touch each other as well) should be heeded and the child placed in a treatment oriented setting.

The Exceptions

Latency* Remission

The exception to this general rule is the child who enjoys a "latency remission" [21]. There are schizophrenic children who, beginning around the sixth year of life, experience a "developmental spurt" during which they virtually overtake their normal peers. The signs of thought disorder in such children then become much more subtle. Perseveration and a tendency to be very rigid and literal-minded persist. The tendency to disorganize when very anxious may also persist, but episodes of disorganization will usually be short-lived and present no serious difficulties to either the child or his teacher. Emotions, with the exception of anxiety and anger, remain constricted. The child however now relates quite "normally" to a number of people including a few of his peers. Beginnings will continue to be difficult for such children, and teachers will need to be able to carry the child through these difficult times.

Such children often have high IQ's (a full scale IQ greater than 120) and are well able to compensate quickly for the small associative errors they continue to make. Although such children are almost as likely to manifest

*This term refers to that phase of a child's psychosexual development which lies between the oedipal phase and the onset of adolescence (approximately ages six to eleven inclusive).

schizophrenia during the late adolescent and adult years as are the children who continuously manifest the symptoms of the disorder, there is at present no certain way of fortifying them, while they are in remission, against the return of the disease. Child-rearing practices which emphasize the importance of gentle self-control and which avoid high pressure, achievement-oriented living (e.g. "you must be the best in the class") will probably be most helpful. A strong ego and a good sense of humour (which is necessary to decrease the child's rigidity) are the surest defences against a disabling return of the disease.

Those who interact with "latency remission" children will need to be sensitive to their motor difficulties, as these persist despite the remission in thought and language dysfunctioning. These children will be unable to compete on the sports field with normal peers. Not infrequently, these boys will select girls or younger children to play with. It is most desirable that the boy's father or a close adult male relative spend extra time with him in order to compensate for the child's feelings about being left out of many "boy" activities. At the first signs of returning psychosis professional consultation and treatment should be sought for such a child.

Children Who Present During the Latency Years
There are rare children (usually boys) who relate normally during the preschool years and who have a history of normal development, but who gradually become more withdrawn and preoccupied during the latency years. The onset of the disease in these children resembles that which has been so commonly observed and described in adolescent-onset schizophrenia, i.e. it is gradual and no major stressor can be identified. Teachers become concerned about this child "underachieving" and

"daydreaming" and often will send for the parents to say "something is bothering him". Usually the child's behaviour is significantly more disturbed at home than in the structured school programme. Many parents have unconsciously been waiting for the "second shoe to fall" (i.e. for someone else to notice that something is wrong with their son). Not only will they not necessarily resist the school's recommendation that a professional consultation is in order, they may very well welcome such a consultation.

Childhood Schizophrenia in Girls

Before puberty, five times as many males as females develop the symptoms of schizophrenia. When females do show symptoms of the disease during childhood, the onset (or at least the time at which professional consultation is sought) is usually later [7] and they tend to develop either the "disorganized" type of schizophrenia or the "paranoid" type; the "undifferentiated" type is rarer. Language appears to be less impaired in the girls than in the boys and the affect tends to be more obviously inappropriate and less noticeably constricted.

Since symptoms are often not noted in females until the school years, they are more frequently initally described as "emotionally disturbed, mildly retarded". However, as they mature, the symptoms of schizophrenia emerge unmistakeably. Retrospective historical data obtained from the parents suggest that, despite late identification, the preschool behaviours of schizophrenic girls are not different from those which have been attributed to preschool schizophrenic boys in earlier chapters of this book.

Onset by Means of Acute Psychosis

Chronic schizophrenia at any age tends to begin in a

slow difficult-to-be-certain-of manner. Only rarely does it have its true beginning in an "acute" psychotic episode. Indeed, even the children who are first admitted to hospital with acute and dramatic symptoms usually have a history of developmental delay not unlike that which has already been described in previous chapters of this book, i.e. a delay in speech and gross motor development.

Acute, dramatic, psychotic behaviour can usually be traced to an emotional trauma, e.g. parental separation or divorce, an assault upon the child, etc. A child with a poor developmental history who suffers an acute psychotic episode is most unlikely to fully recover. In most cases the rest of this child's development will be indistinguishable from that of the children who have been symptomatic from earliest childhood.

Some Salient Points

Preserving Self-Esteem

Every effort should be made during the elementary school years to help the schizophrenic child who does not go into remission to build a positive self-concept. Paradoxically, the closer to the norm the child approaches, the more vulnerable is his self-esteem. Even the child who lives with his family in the community and attends a special needs programme has every opportunity after school hours to compare himself to normal children. High-functioning schizophrenic children quickly develop a keen awareness that they are different. They often verbalize their pain to their families. By eleven or twelve years of age they may begin to express a wish to be dead. At the first sign of painful self-awareness, an empathic psychotherapist should begin working with this child.

The only means available to the teacher and the parents to ease this child's pain is extra time spent developing his strengths. If the schizophrenic child can be taught a skill which will win the admiration of his peers it will do wonders for his self-esteem (many of these children are quite musical and can master a musical instrument such as a guitar with ease). It will be some solace to the schizophrenic child if there is an activity at which he can "shine".

Strengths

Strengths can usually be identified in all but the most disorganized of schizophrenic children. It is an error to attempt to "ban" the child's favourite activity (which usually reflects his strengths) on the theory that it is this preoccupation which is preventing more "normal" behaviour. The wise teacher will use a child's preoccupation to help that child grow. Thus, a six year old's constant preoccupation with maps was used by his teacher to teach him a great deal about geography. In order to do this the teacher had to be willing at times to abandon his own curriculum in favour of the child's current preoccupation. The value of the teacher's flexibility was however proven by the amount the child learned in the next few months.

Decisions such as this, to go along with a child's "craziness", must of course be made on an individual basis. Not all of the preoccupations selected by schizophrenic children lend themselves as readily to expanding the child's knowledge. There are times when a teacher will have to persevere in the attempt to divert the child from a current preoccupation onto one which will encourage the child's cognitive growth.

The teacher of the schizophrenic child must be both creative and patient. The disorders in thought and

language and the heightened sensorium which were
described in the previous chapter persist in all but the few
schizophrenic children who enter a "latency remission"
(although word salad, neologisms and echolalia decrease
rapidly with good treatment). The areas of "strength" are
those which are not dependent upon highly organized
ways of conceptualizing, but which actually *benefit* from
the constantly alert sensory system of the schizophrenic
as well as this child's tendency to fragment all incoming
perceptions. Thus, a six year old schizophrenic child was
judged to be "very bright" when he noted that "each
snowflake is different" while his peers were describing
snow as "soft", "white", "cold", etc., attributes which
he was scarcely able to appreciate (since they related to
the whole, or the context).

A preoccupation with how things are put together
and what makes them operate is commonly observed in
schizophrenic children. These children enjoy taking
things apart and should be helped with the task of learning how to reassemble them. Although short term
memory is often impaired, with repetition the child can
learn how to assemble objects and can master the
mechanics of how they function.*

Psychosexual Development
The timing of psychosexual development in schizophrenic children is unpredictable. A child who has never
masturbated may suddenly begin to do so when the
merest chance awakens his interest in his genitals (e.g. an

---

*The mechanical aptitude of schizophrenic children is first seen in the ease
with which they manipulate puzzles and building blocks, later it can be documented on the Performance section of *WISC-R*, where they will score in the
superior range on the Object Assembly, Picture Arrangement and Block
Design Subtests,[22] and still later it should facilitate the learning of such skills
as electronics and mechanics as the children mature into adult life.

injury, or a pair of pants which are too tight or too loose, etc.). For most schizophrenic children, prior to adolescence, the genitals appear to achieve no special psychological significance, i.e. all parts of their bodies are valued equally (this is most unlike the normal child who is more sensitive and self-conscious about his genitals than about other parts of his body).

Even high-functioning, "normal", latency remission schizophrenic children can be easily persuaded by their peers to expose themselves. Children with psychosexual conflicts may thus exploit the lack of inhibition of the schizophrenic child. Teachers will have to be alert to the possibility of this occurring, particularly with schizophrenic children who are being educated amongst normal peers. The child who has "set up" the schizophrenic child should be identified and disciplined (if appropriate) while the schizophrenic child should receive careful explanations regarding the social inappropriateness of his behaviour and the value attached to privacy.

More About Symptoms and Interventions

Social Norms

During the elementary school years the shaky ego boundary of the schizophrenic child is revealed by his inability to comprehend social norms.* The ease with which this child can be induced to expose himself has already been described. This child will have great difficulty comprehending the need for privacy of those around him. He will stare inappropriately and verbalize aloud

*The Verbal Comprehension score on the WISC-R of even the brightest schizophrenic child is almost always one or more standard deviations *below* the norm (i.e. in the mildly retarded range).

what he sees, interrupt constantly and in most inappropriate ways, talk and laugh aloud when he feels so inclined and regardless of the setting, over-personalize all interactions (i.e. everything which happens relates especially to *him*), approach others uncomfortably closely, and in all matters and at all times demonstrate an inability to integrate social norms. In schizophrenic girls, the social inappropriateness often has a histrionic quality and may be accompanied by much giggling and seductiveness.

Any attempt to explain acceptable public behaviour to a schizophrenic child will be met with a perplexed look and an increase in anxious and disruptive behaviour. The schizophrenic child responds to *internal* wishes and stimuli, not external norms. The most difficult task facing the psychotherapist of the schizophrenic of any age is helping the schizophrenic learn to set aside narcissistic impulses for objective reality [23].

Hallucinations

It is rare for schizophrenic children to hallucinate during the preschool years, although at times even the preschool child appears preoccupied and bursts out with sudden exclamatory remarks apparently "addressed to the air", which cause concerned observers to wonder if the child is responding to a "voice" or to an "apparition".

The actual experience of hallucinations can however be confirmed only in the child who communicates verbally. Schizophrenic children have described for the author "lights on the wall" ("which mommy cannot see") and "ghosts" ("which mommy and daddy say are not there"). Most of these experiences occur at night and prevent the child from sleeping. The child does believe the parent or therapist who says that this experience is not real, however he will continue to protest "but I *can* see it". Television and movies can also stimulate visual hallucinatory experiences in such children (a seven year old described "seeing"a super hero on the author's wall).

It seems likely that at least part of the basis for these hallucinatory experiences can be attributed to the inability of the child to contain thought within himself (the ruptured ego boundary again) coupled with the child's too keen sensorium (even in adolescence, schizophrenics continue to describe their memories as being extraordinarily vivid: "I can still *see* it"). It should be gently pointed out to the child that these "pictures" and "voices" belong *inside* the head (likening the experience to dreams will help the child to understand).

Delusions

The delusions of schizophrenia during the childhood years include those due to overidentification (e.g. "I am an eggplant" after reading a story which featured talking vegetables) and those due to grandiosity (e.g. "I already know all that" in reference to material the child has never before encountered). The best response to delusions is careful and repeated attention to helping the child feel safe with reality (e.g. "Boys are much nicer than eggplants"; "It's all right not to know—you *can* learn").

Sleep Behaviour

The sleep disturbance which is a part of the schizophrenic process is a lifelong problem. The capacity of the child for sleep waxes and wanes unpredictably over the years. During the elementary school years, the child can be taught to remain on his bed and not disturb the rest of the family. Sometimes a "boring" book will help induce sleep. It is best to avoid sedation (since sooner or later the child must find a way of coping with his reduced capacity for sleep).

Still Unpredictable

The schizophrenic child has "good" periods and "bad" periods. Unfortunately, there is usually no easily discernible pattern to his behaviour. Sometimes it seems "he is always most difficult in the spring" but after a few predictable "ups and downs" a "cycle" is interrupted. During times when the child is more in contact with reality and better able to learn, those who work with the child should move in with an accelerated programme. With careful and consistent intervention, as the child matures, the "bad" periods will become shorter and the child himself will start to regulate his moods.

The "Learning Disabled" Schizophrenic Child

The tendency of the schizophrenic child to perseverate can lead to severe difficulties with arithmetical operations. It should be remembered that this child fragments (learns things in pieces) and is resistant to embracing more than one concept at a time. The difficulty of the schizophrenic child in "changing sets" can be seen in activities as diverse as following the action in a fairy tale (wherein the setting of the action may change three or four times within the space of a few paragraphs) or in switching from addition to subtraction to multiplication to division. Once the child becomes accustomed to *adding* numbers, he may be very resistant to learning *other* ways of manipulating these same numbers. To the child, these different ways of manipulating numbers will seem to be a sudden change in the rules, and will arouse great anxiety. A few schizophrenic children may be willing to learn arithmetical operations only *after* some years of performing them on a calculator. Nothing will be achieved by forcing this issue with the anxious perseverative child. We do after all have calculators!

The schizophrenic child does not have a "reading disability" in the truest sense. Most of these children "decode" (read words) with no difficulty whatsoever. Many have learned to read while watching television during the preschool years. There remains however a significant gap throughout the elementary school years between what the child can *read* and what he can *comprehend.*

Schizophrenic children have significant difficulty scanning a page in search of something specific. It may be that this deficit in functioning is due to a disturbance in the functioning of the external eye muscles (the muscles which control the movements of the eye) [24]. Certainly, the children who have a history of crossed eyes appear to have the greatest difficulty with this task. This deficit will not only markedly slow the child's reading, but is certain to dampen his enthusiasm for reading. Coupled with the child's problems with the fragmentation of incoming information and keeping his thoughts focused (every phrase read can trigger a train of associations), the schizophrenic child is most unlikely to read for pleasure. The few such children who do become avid readers, usually read only factual material such as encyclopedias or technical magazines. Only rarely will they elect to read less concrete literature.

Understanding Idiom
The inability of the schizophrenic child to attend to context makes idiomatic speech particularly difficult for this child to understand. One such child reacted to the author's attempts to explain popular usage ("the word means . . . *because* . . .") by interrupting her and shouting "No *because!*". This same child at age eight and a half came up to the author and *hit* her on the shoulder after she had stated "I can't see it because the sun is

hitting the slate''. Careful and patient explanations will ease this problem. It cannot be totally alleviated. The schizophrenic remains a concrete (literal-minded) thinker who has great difficulty accepting that a single word can have multiple meanings.

Some may overcompensate for this deficit later by making a career out of studying semantics. It has also been suggested by teachers that learning a second language will help convince the child that the meaning of a word is not fixed forever in time. Humour, with its frequent play on words, can be most helpful to a schizophrenic child who is not paranoid and who is willing to trust and try to learn. The most difficult child to introduce to humour and to teach an acceptance of popular usage of words is the paranoid child. It can take many years to decrease this child's rigidity, even after the child acquires the rudiments of a sense of humour.

The Therapeutic Alliance

''I must talk sense not nonsense'' was the verbal response of an eight year old schizophrenic child to the sudden appearance of his therapist while he was engaged in bizarre behaviour. This child had become attached to his therapist, and had come to understand that she disapproved of ''nonsense''.

Some ability to reason remains even in the most severely thought disordered schizophrenic. Although the child's ability to *express* affect is severely compromised, some capacity to *feel* remains. When motivated to do so (either by a wish to please or by a wish to achieve) the child can develop an ''observing'' ego (the ability to observe his own behaviour), can form a therapeutic alliance (a working relationship with another for the purpose of psychotherapy), and through these can learn to regulate his own thoughts and behaviour. This alliance will need to be very strong if it is to persuade the child to accept a consensual interpretation of reality in place of his own idiosyncratic view.

Motor Functioning

There will be little change either for the better or for the worse in the schizophrenic child's motor functioning during the elementary school years. Left to himself, this child is very unlikely even to attempt most team sport activities. The advantage of a good gross motor programme is that it will encourage the child to undertake much more complex motor activities than the child would otherwise attempt. The gross motor programme therefore offers the child a unique opportunity to develop the concept of mastery, i.e. when I work at something hard it does get easier.

Gross motor therapy does not appear to increase the child's muscle tone. However, even those children with poor muscle tone can master a great many complex motor activities (such as running, hopping, etc.). One of the major advantages of educating schizophrenic children as a separate group is that it enables them to compete unself-consciously with each other without the threat to gender identity or self-esteem which can result from finding themselves inferior. In a therapeutic milieu only the most paranoid of children will resist involvement with their peers.

Vocations Ahead

By ten to twelve years of age the teachers and the therapists who work with schizophrenic children should begin actively planning for helping the child learn a marketable skill. The child's strengths and interests should have been identified and cultivation of these begun (e.g. art, mechanics, electronics, etc.). The child should have acquired sufficient ego strength to be able to think silently and persist in a difficult task (untreated, these children give up very easily). The child should have some conscious awareness that beginnings are hard, but that the incomprehensible becomes understandable with effort. In short, the child must have at least the beginnings of a concept of mastery, an essential developmental milestone if the child is to live a productive life.

By early adolescence, negativism will be as strong as it was during the preschool years. If the child has not acquired some ability to discipline himself during the elementary school years, puberty will present such major difficulties that pressure may mount upon those who care for this child to institutionalize him permanently.

CHAPTER SIX

ADOLESCENCE

In adolescence it is the developmental task of each of us to define *who* we are and *what* it is we intend to do. Schizophrenic children who have been institutionalized in childhood or who are institutionalized early in adolescence will at best approach this task only at an unconscious level. For those who have, however, received the benefits of a special education and who have lived their childhood years within the community, adolescence brings with it the final challenges which must be met if the individual is to become a productive member of society.

Therapy Please

During the adolescent years psychotherapy is essential to the schizophrenic who has been psychotic since childhood. There are still very few therapists willing to work with psychotics, and many families will have to search with diligence to find an empathic and knowledgeable therapist who has no need to deny the seriousness of the child's illness and who will not seek to attribute all of the child's problems to the family [25] . It is well worth the effort, since if the child is to achieve any of the developmental landmarks of adolescence the child must have an "auxiliary ego" (the role of the therapist) outside of the immediate family.

It is most desirable that therapy begin during the pre-adolescent period, i.e. before pubertal changes have accelerated. As the body begins the process of change, the schizophrenic child's anxiety will escalate. Most schizophrenic children will respond to this increase in anxiety with an increase in withdrawal, isolation, autism (a preoccupation with inner stimuli), and negativism. They are therefore most unlikely to establish a relationship with a psychotherapist after the onset of puberty. If therapy begins before puberty, the therapist can also take an active role in preparing the child cognitively for the physical changes which will attend puberty.

The Body Matures

The extensive bodily changes of puberty have a dramatic impact upon even the most emotionally constricted of childhood schizophrenics. Usually, the immediate reaction is an increase in disorganized behaviour.

"Wet Dreams" and Menarche
It is important to prepare the child well in advance for the occurrence of nocturnal emissions ("wet dreams") or for menarche (the onset of menstruation). Even with careful preparation, the schizophrenic child is particularly prone to reacting to these events by developing enuresis (urinary incontinence) and/or encopresis (fecal incontinence). It is as if the child viewed pubertal events as the loss of his own ability to control his excretions. Careful explanation can help to minimize these regressive responses in most schizophrenic children. A few will require firm behavioural intervention to suppress enuresis and encopresis. Some will show regressive behaviour and refuse to care for themselves adequately only during the menstrual cycle.

Delusions

The schizophrenic child is particularly prone to bodily delusions during the height of pubertal changes. Thus, one fourteen year old boy appeared to respond to his increase in muscle mass by developing the delusion that he was the Incredible Hulk. Clearly, the sudden increase in muscle mass was not the *only* reason he entertained this delusion (the boy was completely unable to verbalize his intense rage against his paranoid alcoholic father), nevertheless his bodily changes added credence to this delusion.

It is not unusual for schizophrenic children to become increasingly preoccupied with internal stimuli during the pubertal years. Thus, one thirteen year old boy expressed constantly the belief that his "tummy giggled". When his therapist showed him that this occurred only when he was hungry (by giving him a glass of milk) his anxiety decreased and he replaced the word "giggled" with the more accurate "gurgled". Another fifteen year old boy complained of his "chest collapsing into his stomach". After some exploration of this fear in psychotherapy it became evident that this delusion expressed the boy's concern that his chest muscles were underdeveloped compared with those of his peers (the boy was of asthenic build).

Hypotonia Again

Schizophrenic adolescents become painfully aware of their physical deficits. Many of the boys spontaneously take up weight lifting or jogging in an effort to improve their muscle development. Some succeed in developing a normal muscle mass, although it cannot be said with certainty whether this is because of the exercise programme they have undertaken or whether this would have happened regardless. Most schizophrenic adolescents who have manifested the symptoms of schizophrenia accompanied by hypotonia since childhood remain under-developed muscularly. Many mature into very asthenic young men. Their skin remains extraordinarily soft (another characteristic of hypotonic childhood schizo-phrenia), further embarrassing their sense of manhood. The girls are of course less troubled by these physical manifestations of the disease, although they may also become preoccupied and concerned regarding their physi-cal strength.*

Awakening Sexuality

In general, the response of the schizophrenic child to increases in genital activity (the increased vaginal secre-tions of girls as well as the nocturnal emissions of boys) is one of fear and disgust. Severely disturbed schizophrenic males have even been observed reacting with terrified self-abuse to a spontaneous erection. This in turn awakens much unconscious anxiety in the teachers and the family of the pubertal schizophrenic. The despair of those who care for the schizophrenic child will never be more intense than during puberty and early adolescence, nor will the pressure for institutionalization ever be greater.

Echopraxia and Delayed Echopraxia

The schizophrenic child and adolescent mimics exact-ly the body movements of others (echopraxia). In severely disturbed youngsters, the child may literally cross his legs when the person opposite him does so and shift his posi-tion in immediate imitation of the person attending him. In the author's experience, much of the schizophrenic

*One adolescent schizophrenic girl obsessed for years regarding the possibil-ity of becoming a wrestler. She made constant efforts to improve her physical strength and inquired repeatedly of her therapist whether she was now "strong enough" to become a lady wrestler (she definitely was not!).

child's early sexual behaviour is at best a "delayed echopraxia", i.e. the youngster imitates the behaviour of his peers rather than acting upon any drive of his own.

The high-functioning schizophrenic child imitates the sexual preoccupations and even the sexual behaviour of his normal peers in fairly obvious ways. Thus, the schizophrenic adolescent will repeat "locker room jokes" without any understanding of what they mean (often confusing the narration and missing the laugh). This teenager may imitate the clothes and mannerisms of his peers in bizarre and inappropriate ways, usually inspiring some rather anxious scapegoating on the part of his peers. If placed in a therapeutic milieu with nonpsychotic peers the schizophrenic youngster is likely to become the object of both their tender concerns and their cruel jokes.

It is not uncommon for the schizophrenic teenager to understand the sexual preoccupation of his peers as meaning that sexuality is the "key to normality". Many a schizophrenic adolescent boy decides that if he can once succeed in sexual intercourse with a girl all of his psychological troubles will be at an end. Similarly, the adolescent schizophrenic female becomes convinced that if she can succeed in "having a boyfriend" it will prove that she is "normal". Given the weak ego boundary of the adolescent schizophrenic, with its accompanying fear of physical penetration, the anxiety of the schizophrenic adolescent is much increased by his or her own conviction that the "key to normality" lies in the achievement of sexual intercourse.

Anhedonia*

The capacity to experience intense pleasure is

*Anhedonia is a Greek term meaning "the absence of pleasure". It has been used in connection with schizophrenia to describe the inability of the schizophrenic to feel pleasure.[25]

impaired in the schizophrenic adolescent. The youngster who has demonstrated the symptoms of schizophrenia since early childhood has begun to "burn out" emotionally. The child is well able to be affectionate and feel a special love for significant individuals in his life. However, the ability to experience joy, spontaneity, pleasure, is either absent or very much decreased. The only emotions besides love and affection which the child appears to be able to experience with any degree of intensity are fear, anxiety, and anger; the "emergency emotions" which appear to dominate the emotional life of the schizophrenic adolescent [26].

The inability to experience pleasure very much colors the sexual experiences of the schizophrenic adolescent. Thus, the increase in sexual drive which attends puberty is experienced by the young schizophrenic as "tension". It appears to totally lack any pleasant associations, tending instead to increase the youngster's aggressive fantasies and behaviour. Many bizarre behaviours may be observed as the youngster attempts to discharge this increase in inner tension and anxiety (e.g. a twelve year old boy retired to his room to build a bomb to blow up his school).

Frequently there is a temporary increase in the secondary symptoms of the disease. Thus, a fourteen year old girl described, with a mixture of excitement and fear, "seeing" Godzilla. During the same hospitalization she repeatedly asserted that she was Donny Osmond's girlfriend (the battle between Donny Osmond and Godzilla for her affections was implicit).

Appropriate masturbation is rarely initiated by such a youngster. Instead, schizophrenic adolescent girls may introduce foreign objects not only into the vagina, but also into other body orifices (e.g. the nose, ears, etc.). It is often during puberty that schizophrenic children who have been educated or institutionalized with the mildly retarded exhibit such bizarre behaviours that they are finally identified as "psychotic".

The Struggle for Identity

"I'm a Girl, a Pearl of a Girl"

With these words, Theodore Rubin described the growing self-awareness of a fictional schizophrenic adolescent [27]. It is the task of the therapist of the schizophrenic child not only to help this child develop a strong sense of self, but to help this child understand that such a sense of self must *precede* a normal heterosexual relationship. The child will resist this, preferring to believe that a sense of identity can be bestowed by means of an interaction with another ("if a boy likes me, I must be a pretty girl"). At times this "passivity" of the schizophrenic adolescent may be so profound that this youngster will look to the external world for everything from a validation of his identity to total physical care. It will require time, patience, and a strong therapeutic alliance before the schizophrenic adolescent will achieve anything approaching an independent sense of self.

It is the need to establish a sense of "being", even vicariously, which can lead to dangerous fantasies and acting out behaviour on the part of the paranoid schizophrenic adolescent. Such adolescents frequently over-identify with public and highly mythologized human beings (e.g. rock groups such as "Kiss", historical figures such as Hitler and Stalin, etc.). If such adolescents are allowed to isolate themselves, and do not confide any of their fantasy material to another human being, the all-too-familiar result is a dramatic newspaper headline announcing that still another paranoid schizophrenic has acted out a grandiose fantasy.

Ambivalence

The normal adolescent re-examines all the important relationships in his life in relation to his rapidly maturing self-concept. For the schizophrenic adolescent this re-examination brings the symptom of *ambivalence* very much to the fore. The schizophrenic adolescent may be so shaken by the age-appropriate attempt to examine his views of himself and his family that whatever ability he may have acquired during childhood to make decisions and exercise judgement may give way during early adolescence to totally disorganized behaviour. In extreme cases the schizophrenic adolescent may even lose the ability to walk without going back and forth several times in an obsessional and ritualistic manner.

The rigidity and literal-mindedness of the schizophrenic adolescent may make any incongruency in the family's value system intolerable to this youngster (for example a forgotten promise which is inadvertently broken, etc.). The struggle to assimilate the most basic of contradictions and ambiguities—which go unnoticed by most teenagers—can result in dramatic love-hate swings in the schizophrenic adolescent accompanied by unpredictable outbursts of rage. It is ambivalence which dictates that every outburst of rage must be followed by an almost equally intense re-affirmation of love.

To Live or Not to Live

Every schizophrenic adolescent who achieves any understanding of external reality and any awareness of his own struggles with psychosis will have to struggle with "why me?". This is the question which assails every human being who must integrate a chronic disability. The risk of suicide is great at this time, as is the risk of violent acting out. Some youngsters cannot tolerate the pain and anxiety of seeing themselves as deficient in any way. They will instead project whatever difficulties they have onto the external environment ("I was fine until Mr. --- embarrassed me in front of all the other kids"; "My mother has always had it in for me, that's why my nerves are bad", etc,). When projection occurs there is always a danger of violent acting out, as the schizophrenic adolescent may seek to destroy that which he believes is preventing him from functioning normally. If suicidal or homicidal ideation cannot be "talked out" in a therapeutic relationship, the schizophrenic adolescent may well require a period of protective hospitalization (sometimes involuntary) to carry him through this crisis.

The Cognitive Spurt

"I Can Learn"

For most childhood schizophrenics puberty brings with it a marked acceleration in cognitive development. Once the shock of acquiring a new body has been integrated, and if the schizophrenic child is in a stable and comfortable living situation, both the child and those who care for him may find a marked improvement in the child's ability to reason. This is a time of very active learning. In an ungraded setting, some of these youngsters will now cover three or four grade levels in a single academic year. This sudden improvement in the ability to master academic material will in turn improve the child's self-esteem. The satisfaction derived from this will very much ease the tensions arising out of the struggle to achieve an identity and sexual maturity.

Intellectualization and Sublimation

The tendency to make an intellectual exercise out of all experience is a highly adaptive defence mechanism used by adolescents to cope with the ever-increasing demands society places upon them. Wise teachers and therapists will help the young schizophrenic adolescent adopt this defence (the schizophrenic youngster is unlikely to develop this defence without some psychotherapeutic input). It is this defence which makes of adolescents a highly critical, difficult to live with group of individuals. It is however also this defence which can help ease the schizophrenic adolescent's pain over his own emotional and thought disturbances. The youngster can be helped to "understand" his illness and even to rationalize the fact that it has endowed him with some special "sensitivity" and heightened awarenesses.

Sublimation is the ability to derive gratification from non-sexual endeavours. It can readily be appreciated that if the schizophrenic adolescent can derive pleasure from such activities as art or music, it will go a long way towards easing the anhedonia previously described.

Leaving Home

If a suitable residential treatment setting is available, adolescence is a most appropriate time for the young schizophrenic to leave home. Separation from home will be a difficult task. Perhaps because he is so vulnerable he clings to his family and they to him. However, during adolescence his own developmental drive favours a move towards independent living and better peer relations. As sexuality increases there is some very age-appropriate tension between the young schizophrenic and his family. It is unlikely the move away from home will ever be any easier.

Ideally, the young schizophrenic should enter an open treatment setting (preferrably a residence within his own community) at sixteen to eighteen years of age. The treatment programme should attach much importance to the work ethic ("you must make your own way in this world") and to helping the residents experience themselves as a part of the community. Group therapy (utilizing peer pressures to disallow psychotic behaviours and social isolation), drama therapy (demonstrating social skills and job interview approaches) and current event groups (interpreting the community to the residents) are treatment approaches which should prove most helpful. Self-pity and self-involvement can also be much attenuated by involving the young schizophrenic with other handicapped individuals. Doing something for others can be an effective means of interrupting the young schizophrenic's total preoccupation with himself.

And Now to Work

It will take many years to prepare a childhood schizophrenic for entering the work force. It is for this reason that the recommendation was made that vocational planning begin as early as ten or eleven years of age. The hypersensitive sensorium, motor slowness and possible weakness, difficulty keeping thoughts in focus, difficulty containing thought and emotion, susceptibility to unreasonable fears and rages, very shaky sense of self (which makes authority figures especially threatening), and inability to note and understand the meaning of context will all create special problems in the work situation. It will require a long and careful training period to insure that the schizophrenic himself understands where the problems lie and is able to regulate his own behaviour. If some care is taken to identify the strengths of each individual and to set up a training programme for each individual, success will often be achieved. The only *sine qua none* is that the schizophrenic adolescent himself must be highly motivated to achieve mastery. All therapy during the adolescent years must have as its major objective the achievement of this motivation.

CHAPTER SEVEN
IN CONCLUSION
The Long Haul

The author is painfully aware that what has been described in the preceding chapters is an illness which interferes significantly with each stage of a child's development. There are no cures, and there are few precautions which can be taken in one stage which will ease the special difficulties encountered in the next. The interventions which have been described can only relieve symptoms, they cannot cure.

It must also be acknowledged that the interventions which have been described depend upon the availability of knowledgeable professionals such as special education teachers, occupational therapists, psychiatrists and clinical psychologists, as well as the existence of small special education classrooms and residential treatment facilities, all of which are community-based. In many communities in North America and Europe neither the professionals nor the facilities which have been described are available.

In the few communities in which such professionals and facilities do exist, it is usually the preference of the community to set aside these resources for children who are far less disturbed than schizophrenic children. On occasion, the highest functioning of schizophrenic children do make their way into treatment facilities where, too often, they are introduced to "acting out" (drug abusing and behaviourally-disturbed) youngsters. It goes without saying that the schizophrenic often begins to imitate the behaviourally disturbed. Thus, every community has its alcohol and drug-abusing young schizophrenics.

Specialized resources for schizophrenic children are expensive. There is no *practical* way that they can become universally available. In a small community, economics will dictate that schizophrenic children will have to be educated with other handicapped children. The real danger in such a community is that the schizophrenic child will be understimulated. Under these circumstances it is best if good resource help can be provided so that the schizophrenic child can remain within the *normal* stream. An understimulated schizophrenic child will either retreat into a fantasy world or become a severe behaviour problem (as the child's energy is diverted into agitated over-activity and anger). Sedation, which will then be offered, is not a solution.

Parent Interest Groups
There are laws in place in both North America and Europe which have recognized the need for improved services to disabled children. If the parents of schizophrenic children will seek out other parents within their own community they will find that not only can they give each other much needed emotional support, but as a group they are more likely to succeed in their efforts to establish community-based treatment programmes for their troubled children. This can of course only occur if the parents "come out of the closet" and view their child's disorder without guilt and without shame. Only when schizophrenia achieves public recognition as the severe and chronic disabler it is will the advantages of 20th Century medicine become as much a part of the treatment of this disease as they are now a part of the treatment of such diseases as

diabetes and muscular dystrophy. This is unlikely to happen until the families of schizophrenics organize themselves and make this demand.

It is suggested that the parents who undertake to organize parent interest groups welcome to their midst the parents of adult schizophrenics. In some situations they might join groups of relatives and friends of adult schizophrenics. This will make it far easier for the parents of schizophrenic children not only to accept realistically that their child is suffering from a lifelong disorder, but also to enlist the help of existing mental health agencies. If the parents are to establish residences in the community for their children as they reach late adolescence the assistance of established mental health agencies will be invaluable. It is important that parents appreciate early that there will be pressure to institutionalize the schizophrenic child as the child matures. In fact, the brighter, more high-functioning schizophrenic children often have more dramatic psychotic symptoms as they grow older and are more likely to be candidates for provincial or state hospitals than are the more severely affected, lower-functioning schizophrenic children who have considerably less energy and are often far less of a problem to society.

Denial
Perhaps the most disabled schizophrenic child of all is the one whose family needs to deny the nature of the child's disturbance. The author has seen families who will seek until they find a doctor who will tell them that their child is primarily mentally retarded (in preference to a diagnosis of mental illness). The opposite extreme can also be seen, the family that is certain that all of their child's emotional and thought disturbances are a consequence of being a ''gifted'' child with a ''motor disturbance'' or a ''learning disability''. Without treatment, the

child from either type of family is likely to be eventually institutionalized, the former with the mentally retarded, the latter with the mentally ill.

The Mildly Affected

The children who have been described in this book can be viewed as moderately to severely affected by the disease. There are children who follow the same developmental course and manifest the same developmental disabilities, but are far less disabled. Such children are usually placed in classes for the "language disabled" or in "slow learner" groups. In a few cases either the child's symptoms are so mild or the family's tolerance for deviation is so great that the child is not identified at all. Teachers will often advise the family to seek professional consultation, but will not press the family when the family fails to do so. In many cases children such as these remain within the regular classroom. They are the "quiet loner" whom every teacher of elementary school has seen.

It has long been known that those who present with the symptoms of mental illness during the adolescent years and who remain chronically mentally ill frequently have a long history of both poor school performance and poor peer relations [28]. Children such as these could also benefit greatly from the type of therapeutic interventions which have been recommended in this book. Unfortunately, it may be many years before the community will be willing to set aside enough funding to allow all "at risk" children to benefit from small classrooms and intensive therapeutic input.

"It's Untreatable"

Most mental health professionals regard schizophrenia as "untreatable". Indeed, many who will read this book will even take it as a confirmation of that view. It must however be stressed that "incurable" does not mean "untreatable". There are many chronic illnesses which are at present incurable but which nevertheless receive the best of treatment that modern medicine can provide. It is this "best of treatment" for which this book pleads. We have long known that there are a sizable number of "ambulatory" schizophrenics, that is, schizophrenics who function quite well in our society despite a tendency to be socially isolated ("loners") and to think in an idiosyncratic manner. The goal of all treatment of schizophrenia should be to achieve at least such a state of function.

Pharmacotherapy

Very little has been said in this book regarding the use of major tranquilizers. The reason for that is that there is a good deal of evidence that in childhood-onset schizophrenia they are of little benefit. The medications which are presently available for the treatment of schizophrenia are excellent at alleviating paranoid delusions, auditory hallucinations, acute anxiety states, and severe sleep disturbance. The author did advocate the use of a sedative for the severe sleep disturbance of very young schizophrenic children. Major tranquilizers are also most usefull in adolescence when the childhood schizophrenic may develop many secondary symptoms of the disease such as hallucinations and delusions.

The author is not opposed to the use of major tranquilizers, but advocates that they be used very cautiously and only if there can be an observable relief in symptoms. They should *not* be used in order to make a child compliant and therefore "no trouble" to an environment which is in fact harmful to the child. If medications are used in combination with positive environmental manipulation and a constant attention to the milieu in which the child is growing and developing, and with specific target symptoms in mind, they can be most helpful.

Medications rarely relieve the hallucinations of childhood. The best intervention is to teach the child to ignore them and even to "look away" (since they are usually visual). This advice to ignore and refuse to "look at" visual hallucinations also has proven most helpful with schizophrenic adolescents. It should be tried before major tranquilizers are used, unless there are other reasons (such as severe paranoid delusions) for using major tranquilizers.

Other Siblings

Perhaps the most difficult task facing the parents of a schizophrenic child is maintaining the mental health of the "normal" siblings of a schizophrenic child while the schizophrenic child remains within the nuclear family. If good treatment facilities are available for the child and psychotic behaviours are dealt with firmly and early in development, the childhood years may pass relatively uneventfully. Parents should be cautious however about placing too much responsibility upon normal siblings for looking after the schizophrenic child. One of the significant advantages of family support groups is that the siblings of the schizophrenic child also derive benefit from such groups (by meeting other siblings who have shared their fate). In adolescence, it has already been advocated that an effort be made to place the schizophrenic youngster in a residence in the community. This will benefit everybody, the schizophrenic adolescent, the siblings of such an adolescent, and the parents of such an adolescent. As long as the residence is in the community the schizophrenic adolescent can maintain close contact with his family. The other siblings will now have a chance to experience a "normal family life" [25].

In Conclusion

There can be joy in raising a schizophrenic child. These children can return love, often in the most unexpected and surprising ways. They can be generous and thoughtful and highly creative. There is also a special satisfaction in watching someone develop who has been able to do so only with difficulty. It is this special satisfaction which can help carry the families and those who work with schizophrenic children through the long intervals of time when no progress seems to be achieved.

Little has been said about research, but research there must be. Research is in fact an inevitable consequence of acceptance into the mainstream of medicine. The greatest impediment to research into the causes of mental illness has been the isolation of the affected population in state and provincial hospitals which are far removed from university medical centres. The acceptance of schizophrenic children into the community and into community-based children's hospitals will insure that a group of scientists will arise whose major passion will be to find a solution to the riddle of mental illness. Indeed, even as this book goes to press, a marked acceleration is already in evidence in research into the causes of the *dementias*. One of the major functions of parent interest groups should be to demand and support an increase in such research.

TO THE PHYSICIAN

TO THE PHYSICIAN

By far the majority of schizophrenic children will first be seen by a pediatrician or a family physician. Most families will instinctively begin by consulting their primary care physician. The physician thus consulted has a rare opportunity to help the family develop a positive attitude toward their child's disability.

The First Three Months
In the few cases where schizophrenia is already manifesting itself at birth, the infant is a "floppy" infant. The severely affected have a poor suck and are lethargic, sleepy babies. The examining physician will find very poor muscle tone and may note (often by four weeks) an unusual alertness to visual stimuli in an otherwise lethargic infant. There are no other signs of neurological dysfunction (the EEG will be normal), although the physician may also be able to document the baby's tendency to prefer twirling objects to the human face. If such information is available, a family history of mental illness or mental retardation should further raise the physician's index of suspicion.

Feeding is a potential source of much stress to this parent-child relationship. The lethargic infant does not feed well. Poor suck may make it impossible to breastfeed this baby. Many mothers will experience the child's feeding difficulties as a keen sense of personal failure. The physician can do so much to strengthen the bond between mother and child merely by anticipating for the troubled parent the consequences of the child's motor problem.

Six Months to Two Years

Between six months and eighteen months signs of the schizophrenic process make their appearance even in infants who are not yet significantly hypotonic. Primitive adaptive reflexes persist while the more age-appropriate reflexes are slow to develop. (Techniques for performing the necessary developmental examinations are well described in the literature [29],[30].) The physician will need to examine for the persistance of immature reflexes since the actual motor milestones are not reliable indicators of intact development in a schizophrenic child (most preschizophrenic infants will hold their heads on time, sit on time, and walk on time). A child who avoids sitting unsupported (and routinely props himself on tables or against walls) is a cause for concern. Visual alertness in the presence of lethargic motor activity is also a cause for concern (the child who "looks" but is slow to reach).

It is often toward the end of the first year of life or the beginning of the second year of life that frequent wakefulness becomes the "presenting complaint". If the child is walking and can get out of the crib (fortunately most of these children cannot) the risk of injury may also then become an issue.

The Two Year Old

Between two and three years of age the slow development of language becomes the parents' chief concern. More than seventy-five percent of preschizophrenic two year olds will show speech delay. Moreover, the preschizophrenic two year old often prefers letters, numbers, calculators, etc. to the stuffed animals and noisy mobile toys which the normal two year old cherishes. The perseverative tendency of the preschizophrenic two year old makes it all too easy for this youngster to slip into spending many hours viewing television. The echoing of television commercials may appear as the child's only language in the third year of life (other than the naming of a few objects needed daily such as "milk", "cookie", etc.). The examining physician can note motor mannerisms and facial grimacing in the preschizophrenic two year old, as well as a growing motor agitation. The family now describes much difficulty falling asleep in addition to the frequent wakefulness during the night.

The Three Year Old

By three years of age the examining physician can observe and document the following signs and symptoms of hypotonic childhood schizophrenia [10] : hypotonia, macrocephaly (a head circumference greater than the 75th percentile), a head circumference which is large relative to the child's height, lax joints, an abnormal head shape (either brachycephaly or dolichocephaly), hypercanthism, short fingers (a mid-finger to hand length ratio less than the 25th percentile) in the presence of long hands (a hand length greater than the 75th percentile), a prominent nasal bridge, unusually deep-set eyes, the persistence of soft velvety skin (resembling that of a newborn infant), decreased muscle mass, decreased muscle power, and reflexes in the upper limbs which are either markedly decreased relevant to those in the lower limbs or totally unobtainable. The presence of strabismus, lordosis, flat feet, poor ability to chew (which may later emerge as an articulation defect), unusual pallor, and dilated pupils should all further increase the physician's index of suspicion. Finally, this child will have marked difficulty mastering stairs, especially going down, and will be late in selecting a hand preference (handedness may not be determined until the child is six to eight years of age). Table 1 itemizes the signs and symptoms of schizophrenia in childhood.

Other than speech delay, the most frequent complaints the parents of the preschizophrenic will present to a physician are phobic behaviour ("He is so terrified of insects, I can't put him outside"), difficulty falling asleep, unexplained and very prolonged periods of upset in an otherwise "good" child, "fussy eating", frequent wakefulness, and a strange kind of persistence (perseveration). It is important that the physician be alert to receiving these complaints, since mothers are often very ambivalent about voicing complaints and fears about a child who seems so very "good".

The poor judgement of the schizophrenic toddler presents major problems to the child's caretakers. It is most difficult to protect these children from accidental trauma, since they are so slow to learn from experience and even slower to master enough language to be able to understand verbal warnings. Occasionally, hyperactivity also appears during the second year of life, adding still another dimension of danger. If this child is also wakeful, then there is a significant risk that the child will injure himself during the night (the author knows of one such youngster who broke eight harnesses designed to keep him in his crib before he was three, and who once pulled a mix-master down upon himself in the middle of the night).

Table 1:

*Signs and Symptoms of Schizophrenia in Childhood [7,10]

Physical Characteristics	*Symptoms*
Hypotonia	Blunted Affect
Brachycephaly or	Perseveration
Dolichocephaly	Inappropriate Affect
Long Hands (>75%)	High Anxiety
Decreased Muscle Power	Fragmented Thought
Decreased Muscle Mass	Hyperacusis
Hyporeflexia	Monotonous Speech
Hypercanthism	Loose Associations
Soft Velvety Skin	Neologisms
Head > Height	Echolalia
Increased Head	Illogicality
Circumference (>75%)	Mannerisms
Prominent Nasal Bridge	Grimacing
Deep-set Eyes	Perplexity
Short Fingers	Autism
($\frac{\text{mid finger}}{\text{hand length}}$ <25%)	Clang Associations
	Incoherence
Lax Elbows	
Lax Metacarpal/Phalangeal	
and Wrist Joints	

*No child will manifest *all* of the above. A minimum of seven of the physical characteristics and nine of the symptoms is required to make a positive diagnosis.

Associated Signs	*Associated Symptoms*
Lordosis	Paranoia
Strabismus	Ambivalence
Articulation Defect	Delusions
Flat Feet	Hallucinations
Loss of Flexor Tone	Poverty of Speech
No Arm Swing When Walking	Poverty of Content of
Abnormal Gait	Speech
Dilated Pupils	Talking to Self
Mixed Dominance	Hoarding
Pallor	Motor Agitation
	Sleep Disturbance

The physician who has known the preschizophrenic child since birth will not be surprised when this child fails to develop speech by three years of age. In the presence of all the signs which have been described, in particular the motor signs (autistic children, many of whom remain mute, do not usually have these motor signs), the physician can assure the parents that speech will develop (all schizophrenic children develop speech). It is however desirable to warn the parents that even when the child does speak it may remain difficult to understand him since disordered thought processes are likely to be revealed by the child's speech. Many parents of schizophrenic children convince themselves that as soon as their child talks the entire developmental nightmare will be at an end. It is therefore important that physicians make some effort to help parents anticipate the next stage in the child's development

Since schizophrenic children consistently surmount developmental obstacles (the child is slow to relate, but the child *does* eventually relate, the child is slow to learn, but the child *does* learn, etc.) the parents of schizophrenic children may continue to cherish the hope that the next developmental delay will be the last and that their child will be "normal". It is important to warn the parents against delaying the recommended enrollment of the child in a good therapeutic facility because they anticipate the child's imminent achievement of "normality". Such a delay can harm the child's cognitive development.

The Nursery School and Kindergarten Years
Most children who will manifest schizophrenia in the preschool years have displayed the signs and symptoms described above. Very rarely, a child who has developed quite normally and shown no signs of poor motor functioning will begin to show such signs, as well as thought problems, between three and five years of age. In such children, the first signs of the disease are usually high anxiety, perseveration, preoccupation with internal stimuli, wakefulness, and delays in gross and fine motor development. Signs of thought disorder (such as loosening of association) come later, and in many paranoid schizophrenic children are not very prominent symptoms at this young age.

Negativism and hyperactivity now become prominent symptoms in the schizophrenic child. This hyperactivity is quite different from that of the nonschizophrenic hyperactive child. The differential diagnosis is important, since the psycho-active agents which are recommended for use in the true hyperkinetic child can greatly exacerbate the psychotic symptoms of a schizophrenic child. The overactivity of the schizophrenic child is truly aimless and non-goal directed. Most often the child's movements are stereotyped and perseverative, including such activities as rapid pacing, jumping up and down on one spot, dashing about the room making noises, etc. Such over-activity in the presence of the physical signs and symptoms already described should alert the examining physician to avoid all psycho-active stimulants (e.g. ritalin and amphetamines). If the child's over-activity persists and interferes with sleep, an attempt at night time sedation is recommended. Placement of the child in a special preschool programme during the day-time hours will not only alleviate much of the stress upon the parents (who will need some relief from taking care of this child if they are not to "burn out") but will also give highly-trained personnel a chance to interrupt the child's motor stereotypies and stimulate the child's language and social development.

Associated Symptoms

The schizophrenic child tends to run very high fevers even with minor disorders. The parents should be instructed as soon as the disease is suspected regarding the desirability of cooling the child through bathing (in the hope that febrile convulsions can be avoided). Dental caries are commonly observed in such children. No matter how much fuss the child makes, fluoridation and regular dental care are therefore recommended.

If the child has many signs of cholinergic dysfunctioning (e.g. dilated pupils, decreased saliva, very poor muscle tone) it is probably wise to avoid premedication with atropine if anesthesia is needed. It is also prudent to avoid treating enuresis in such children with tricyclics.

Finally, in the rare schizophrenic child who develops a seizure disorder (usually close to puberty) efforts to control the seizures may be frustrated by an exacerbation of the psychotic symptoms. A choice may have to be made between "the lesser of two evils".

Elementary School

Psychosis in many children with a long history of motor and developmental delay may be missed by those who interact with them. This occurs primarily because the most severely affected children have so much language and motor dysfunction that it is only when they have achieved some degree of linguistic fluency that the child's disturbed thought processes are readily appreciated. Thus, the puzzled parents of such a child may appear in a pediatrician or primary physician's office when the child is six and describe a long history of language intervention and motor intervention. The parents will often say "he used to . . . and he used to . . ." and "he no longer . . . but now . . .". This is most likely to occur if the parents have encountered professionals who have observed and treated only certain deficits. The parents are now dismayed and puzzled to find that they still have a most "unusual" child.

The primary care physician may also encounter children at six or seven years of age whose parents deny a history of any problems with motor development and generally insist that the child's development has been totally normal (or even precocious) prior to the present onset of bizarre language and behaviour. Not infrequently these children are identified by a kindergarten or grade 1 teacher and the parents are advised to seek professional assistance. If the child and the family are unknown to the physician, the physician may find photographs of the child revealing. Not infrequently such photographs depict a very "floppy" child, despite parental insistence that the child was "normal".

Most of the children in whom psychosis is truly beginning at this age will manifest the signs and symptoms of *paranoid* schizophrenia (with organized delusions and hallucinations) rather than those of a *disorganized* subtype of schizophrenia. The child who first manifests symptoms of psychosis at this age is often extremely fearful, so that the most prominent symptom is high anxiety, expressed through very inappropriate affect (such as giggling) or poorly masked by multiple obsessional rituals. On physical examination this until-recently normal child will have many of the signs already described, although the hypotonia may be quite mild. Sophisticated tests of motor functioning (such as the Bruinincks-Oseretsky test of neuromuscular proficiency [31] which measures such abilities as running speed and agility, balance, bilateral coordination, etc.) do nevertheless detect a deficit in gross motor functioning in these children as well.

Most female childhood schizophrenics will present between the ages of six and ten. They are frequently initially believed to be "slow learners" or "extremely neurotic" children because of their very high anxiety level. In females, severe disorganization may occur even at this age and even in those who have no previous history of developmental disturbance.

The Role of the Primary Care Physician

The physician in whom the family places its trust can help insure that the family will not be so disrupted by the disturbed child that other "normal" children in the family will be neglected or traumatized. Since it is the primary care physician who first sees the schizophrenic infant or child, it is this physician who must either comply with the family's expressed wish for a referral to a child development or a mental health centre or convince the family which has not made such a request to accept such a referral. The manner in which the first physician who sees the psychotic child interprets the psychosis to the child's family is critical to the family's future attitude towards that child and his illness.

The bond between the schizophrenic child and his parents has often been severely strained by both the child's seeming indifference and the child's psychotic behaviour. The primary care physician can do so much to support the family over the most difficult moments. It is important the physician *never* say "you're managing very well" when the family is showing signs of stress. The family may feel belittled and misunderstood by this approach and is likely to believe the physician does not know anything about what it is like to live with such a child. The more constructive approach is to praise the family, saying "I really don't know how you do it" to which the family is likely to reply, "he's really not that bad".

The more primary care physicians become persuaded that it is important to support both the schizophrenic child and that child's family as the child grows and develops towards maturity, the easier it will be to maintain such children within the community. The caring physician can become a strong advocate for the family as they attempt to set in place optimal educational and residential facilities for their schizophrenic child.

A GLOSSARY OF
SELECTED TERMS

The terms which have been selected for inclusion in this glossary are those which (a) occur frequently in clinical reports describing schizophrenia; and (b) require more elaborate discussion than could have been provided within the context of this book. Terms which have been described within the text in some detail have been excluded from this glossary. The "Psychiatric Dictionary" of Hinsie and Campbell was used in preparing the glossary [32].

AFFECT This refers to the feeling tone accompanying an idea or a thought. In descriptions of the schizophrenic process the word affect is preceded by such qualifying adjectives as *constricted, inappropriate,* or *flat.* References are frequently made to an "affective range", a phrase which refers to the capacity of human beings to express degrees of feeling (e.g. sadness can be expressed in degrees which range from a sad face to full outbursts of crying).

Qualifying adjectives such as *constricted* or *blunted* refer to the fact that in schizophrenia the *range* of human emotions is much reduced (extremes of affective expression persist; it is the middle range which is missing). This reduction in affective expression may continue for some years before the complete ability to express affect is lost.

110

The absence of affective expression is referred to as *flat affect*. (See also BURN OUT.)

Inappropriate affect describes the tendency of schizophrenics to smile or laugh while describing hostile or angry feelings, to look perplexed or sad when describing something which is exciting or might give joy, etc. It is applied to any affective expression which is incongruent with the thought or idea under discussion.

ASTHENIC A term presently used to describe an individual with poorly developed musculature and little body fat. This appearance is accentuated if the individual is also tall.

AUTISM A term first used by Eugen Bleuler to describe the preoccupation of schizophrenics with internal stimuli and subjective wishes. The external environment and objective reality are of secondary importance to the chronic schizophrenic.

The term was also selected by Kanner to designate a group of children whom he believed might represent the earliest form of schizophrenia[5] and whom he labelled "Infantile Autism". The current criteria for diagnosing "Infantile Autism" are:[8](a) onset before 30 months of age; (b) pervasive lack of responsiveness to other people; (c) gross deficits in language development; (d) if speech is present, peculiar speech patterns; (e) bizarre responses to various aspects of the environment; (f) *absence* of delusions, hallucinations, loosening of associations and incoherence as in schizophrenia.

BILATERAL COORDINATION This refers to the ability of the individual to coordinate the movements of the right and left side of the body and the upper and lower limbs.

Children are slow to develop this ability, so that the deficit in functioning which is a part of the childhood schizophrenic's gross motor deficiency is not fully appreciated until the childhood schiozphrenic is nine or ten years of age. The earliest signs of this disability are the failure to transfer objects from one hand to the other (normally achieved by ten to twelve months), a delay in the development of laterality, an "inability to cross the mid-line" (that is the child will pick up objects that are placed on the right side of the body with the right hand and objects which are placed on the left side of the body with the left hand) and the failure to coordinate arm swing during normal walking.

BIOCHEMISTRY This is the science which deals with the chemistry of living organisms. The complexity of living systems has made of this a science quite independent of physical chemistry and organic chemistry, even though the laws of physical chemistry and organic chemistry are fundamental to biological systems.

BIZARRE An adjective used to describe extremely deviant behaviour. The term is essentially synonomous with psychotic.

BURN OUT A term associated with schizophrenia in two ways, the disease process itself, and the effect the afflicted individual has upon those in his or her environment.

The term "burn out" is generally used in reference to the schizophrenic who has been ill for many years and who no longer demonstrates the more dramatic psychotic symptoms such as hallucinations, delusions, high anxiety, motor agitation, etc. By definition the affect in "burned out" schiozphrenics is *flat*. Many "burned out" schizophrenics live in the community and maintain that they are "cured" (although thought disorder, poor judgement and defective ego boundary persist).

"Burn out" in those who care for schizophrenics refers to the tendency of those who work with the chronically mentally ill to lose their enthusiasm, their creativeness, and begin to feel and express hopelessness regarding the schizophrenic individual's ability to cope and function.

CONCRETE THINKING The tendency of the schizophrenic individual to insist upon the most specific and literal meaning of words, ideas, and feelings. In extreme cases a schizophrenic individual may become anxious and agitated if even the simplest attempt is made to elaborate upon an idea or a theme. Concretization is considered to be a part of the association deficit which is a primary symptom of schizophrenia.

CONDENSATION The compression of more than one idea or several words into a single thought or word. The tendency of the schizophrenic to fragment facilitates this process. It is probable that neologisms are actually condensations, i.e. they are fragments of words which have been compressed into a single word which no longer makes sense to anyone including the individual who uses the neologism.

CONGENITAL A medical adjective which means inborn, i.e. a congenital defect is one which is present at birth.

CONSENSUAL VALIDATION A term used by Harry Stack Sullivan to describe the act of comparing one's own thought or feeling about another or about a situation with the thoughts and feelings of others about the same situation. See also *reality testing*.

DEMENTIA A Latin term referring to the loss of the ability to be rational. The original medical term for schizophrenia was *dementia praecox,* a term favored by Kraepelin[33], meaning precocious dementia (a reference to the fact that the schizophrenic process resembled the demented state of the aged).

DEVELOPMENTAL Many theories have been devised to describe the process by which an infant matures into an adult. Thus, there are developmental theories which describe cognitive development, emotional development, psychosexual development, etc. The developmental approach in psychiatry is one which describes the individual in terms of a particular aspect of human development.

EGO A Latin term literally meaning "I", used in psychoanalytic theory to identify that part of the mind which is the mediator between the person and reality. Most theories which address themselves to a dynamic explanation of the schizophrenic process agree that the ego is extremely defective in the schizophrenic individual.

In order to explain the difference between an individual's perception of "self" and "not self" the term "ego boundary" was devised. In normal individuals the ability to distinguish oneself from others and from one's environment is never in question. In schizophrenics the tendency to lose one's sense of self at the slightest challenge is a constant source of trouble. Thus, schizophrenics over-identify with almost every philosophy or idealogy they encounter, e.g. a normal individual reads about the prophets, a schizophrenic is very prone to beginning to think of himself as a prophet! Even after a schizophrenic has made major therapeutic gains and has begun to demonstrate some ability to control disorganized thought processes the deficit in ego boundary continues to interfere with the ability to function in a consistent way.

The term "observing ego" is used to describe that part of an individual's mind which can observe one's own behaviour. Until the schizophrenic can develop this much needed objectivity, psychotherapy is not possible. Therefore, the therapist must focus upon helping the schizophrenic acquire this capacity for self-observation before true therapy can begin.

The term "auxiliary ego" is used to describe the way in which those who seek to interrupt the psychotic process interact with the schizophrenic individual, i.e. an external self (a teacher, an occupational therapist, a psychotherapist, etc.) provides external controls which help regulate the schizophrenic individual until such time as the schizophrenic can master self-regulation.

FINE MOTOR That part of the motor system which involves very complex, finely controlled activity, usually mediated by small muscle groups (in man, this essentially refers to the small muscle groups of the hand). This system is only minimally impaired in most schizophrenic children, although as a result of difficulty stabilizing the trunk and shoulder girdle (gross motor) they may initially experience moderate difficulty with writing.

GENDER IDENTITY This term refers to the subject's concept of sexual identity, rather than the sexual identity itself, i.e. a male may perceive himself as feminine (in which case his gender identity would be female while his sexual identity was male). In schizophrenics gender identity is particularly fragile. The difficulty the male schizophrenic child experiences with group sports and with competition renders the masculine identity of the schizophrenic child most vulnerable.

GRANDIOSITY A term which describes the tendency to over-value oneself. The shaky identity of the schizophrenic youngster results in swings between very grandiose concepts of one's own ability and the opposite extreme. Thus, it is not uncommon to have the same child state within the space of one half of an hour, "I can do anything" and "I can never do anything right". A grandiose fixation can be extremely dangerous as the schizophrenic individual decides to behave outside the limits of all the rules of society. Fixation at the opposite extreme of extremely impoverished self-esteem can lead to a profound inability to function.

GRIMACE Distorted facial expressions (or grimacing) are very common in childhood-onset schizophrenia. They are most often seen when the child is concentrating on a difficult task, be it cognitive or motor. Perplexity (q.v.) also leads to facial grimacing.

GROSS MOTOR That part of the motor system usually mediated by the large muscle groups, such as the long muscles of the arms and legs. It is this system, which controls such activities as walking, running, hopping, etc., which is the most defective in schizophrenic children.

HYPERACUSIS A term which describes the inability of the schizophrenic child to screen out irrelevant sounds.

IDIOSYNCRATIC An adjective used to describe behaviour or thought which deviates mildly to moderately from societal norms. At times such thought and behaviour is now regarded as being on a continuum with psychosis. Usually it passes as a variant of normal.

ILLOGICALITY This term is currently defined as a way of thinking in which conclusions are reached that are clearly erroneous, given the initial premises [7]. The deviation must be dramatic to be considered significant.

INSTITUTIONALIZATION A term used to describe the behaviour of individuals who have spent many years in a custodial environment, totally lacking in stimulation. Children placed in such an environment must inevitably become secondarily mentally retarded since normal cognitive development can occur only in the presence of adequate cognitive stimulation.

NARCISSISM This term is used to describe the tendency of the schizophrenic to worry about ("love") themselves above all others. This preoccupation with self should not be confused with self-esteem, which refers to the *value* one assigns to oneself. Narcissism is generally invoked to explain the terror the schizophrenic expresses in connection with bodily injury (this terror is seen only prior to "burn out". The "burned out" schizophrenic has no fear of pain or injury.) and is often used interchangeably with autism to refer to the schizophrenic's preoccupation with his own wishes.

NEGATIVISM This is a term which refers to the tendency of the schizophrenic child to do the opposite of what he is asked to do. It is an exaggeration of the normal negativism of the preschool years. Again in adolescence, the negativism of the schizophrenic adolescent is an exaggeration of a normal developmental trait. It is characteristic of the schizophrenic child and adolescent to initially respond negatively to requests and suggestions. Often, provided anxiety is not excessive, the child will subsequently comply.

PERPLEXITY This term refers to the state of puzzlement frequently observed in young schizophrenics. The young schizophrenic will often respond to social norms, emotional demands, and abstract ideation with a puzzled frown. If the situation is one in which the child or adolescent experiences much pressure to comprehend, grimacing and motor mannerisms may accompany the perplexed response.

POVERTY OF SPEECH This phrase refers to the tendency of some schizophrenics to reply to all questions with brief phrases or even monosyllables. It will require many questions to illicit any amount of information from a schizophrenic who manifests poverty of speech. In such an individual there is little or no spontaneous communication other than communication which is required to satisfy a need.

PROJECTION This term is used to describe the process of attributing one's own ideas, wishes, or feelings to another. This may be done for the purpose of wish fulfillment (e.g. if an individual very much wishes to be contacted by another individual, he may express this wish as "He wants me to call so I had better call him.") or to relieve unpleasant affects such as fear (e.g. if an individual very much fears another person he may instead state that the other person fears him). Projection is regarded as the mechanism involved in all paranoia. Children project observations, wishes, etc. onto toys and by means of manipulating these toys acquire a degree of mastery (this is termed "projective play"). As a defence mechanism (e.g. to relieve anxiety) projection is usually maladaptive and does not allow for the resolution of a conflict; as a play mechanism projection is usually adaptive. Schizophrenics, unfortunately, tend to use projection as a defence mechanism and tend to avoid projective play.

PSYCHOSEXUAL DEVELOPMENT This refers to the psychoanalytic theory which conceptualizes the process by which human sexuality matures. Freud postulated six stages of psychosexual development, the *oral, anal, genital, oedipal, latency,* and a final resolution of the oedipal conflict during *adolescence.* [34] The sexual drive of the chronic schizophrenic child and adolescent appears to be inhibited so that an orderly progression of psychosexual development is not evident. Some theorists believe that in schizophrenia the process of psychosexual development is arrested in the oral phase, the very first phase of development.

REALITY TESTING This is a term applied to a fundamental ego function, namely the evaluation of the objective world. The ability to perform this function depends upon sensory perception, memory, and an intact ego boundary.

As a result of an impaired ego boundary, projection and paranoia (which is viewed as a projective mechanism) usually replace accurate reality testing in young schizophrenics. The auxiliary ego (or therapist) is essential to the young schizophrenic. In the early stages of therapeutic intervention the "auxiliary ego" will have to do most of the reality testing for the childhood schizophrenic. Later, in a good therapeutic alliance, the child will begin to reality test more accurately on his own.

REGRESSION The term regression refers to a return to an earlier developmental stage. Young schizophrenics are extremely vulnerable to regression. At times therapy with such a child seems to be "one step forward, two steps backwards". Usually regressions are minimal and short-lived. Puberty and early adolescence are the most vulnerable time for the young schizophrenic. Rapid regression to early childhood is often accompanied by acute exacerbations of psychosis during the period immediately following genital maturation and the "growth spurt".

RIGIDITY see CONCRETE THINKING

RITUALISTIC BEHAVIOUR Preschool schizophrenic children often engage in "ritual making" behaviour as they attempt to organize everything from play to daily routine into repetitive behavioural sequences. Usually the child will not carry these rituals to the point of exhaustion. In this, these rituals differ from obsessive compulsive behaviour. The rituals really appear to be the child's effort at organizing his daily experiences.

STEREOTYPY A stereotypy is a repetitive motor behaviour, e.g. rocking back and forth. The term is also applied to posturing, i.e. the maintenance of a given position for a prolonged period of time, and to repetitive play behaviour.

SYNDROME A syndrome is a collection of symptoms which together are believed to be indicative of a disease.

REFERENCES

[1] Rutter, Michael: "Childhood Schizophrenia Reconsidered." *Journal of Autism and Childhood Schizophrenia* 2(4): 315, 1972.

[2] Bleuler, Eugen: Dementia Praecox oder Gruppe der Schizophrenien. In *Handbuch der Psychiatrie* edited by G. Aschaffenburg, Deuticke, Leipzig, 1911.

[3] Bleuler, Eugen: *Textbook of Psychiatry*. Translated by A.A. Brill. Reprint Edition, Arno Press, N.Y., N.Y., 1976.

[4] Schneider, K.: 'Primare und Sekundare Symptome bei Schizophrenie". *Fortschr. Neurol. Psychiatr.* 25:487, 1957.

[5] Kanner, L.: "Autistic Disturbances of Affective Contact". *Nerv. Child* 2:217, 1943.

[6] Fish, B.: The Recognition of Infantile Psychosis in *Modern Perspectives in the Psychiatry of Infancy* edited by J.G. Howells, Brunner/Mazel, N.Y., N.Y., 1979.

[7] Cantor, S., Evans, J., Pearce, J. and Pezzot-Pearce, T.: "Childhood Schizophrenia: Present But Not Accounted For". *Amer. Jour. of Psychiatry* 139(6),1982.

[8] *Diagnostic and Statistical Manual of Mental Disorders*. American Psychiatric Association, Washington, D.C., 1980.

[9] DeMeyer, Marian K.: *Parents and Children in Autism.* V.H. Winston & Sons, Washington, D.C., 1979.

[10] Cantor, S., Pearce, J., Pezzot-Pearce, T. and Evans, J. "The Group of Hypotonic Schizophrenics". *Schizophrenia Bulletin* 7(1) 1, 1981.

[11] Fish, B.: "Neurobiologic Antecedents of Schizophrenia". *Archives of General Psychiatry* 34:1297, 1977.

[12] Bender, L.: "Childhood Schizophrenia: A Clinical Study of 100 Schizophrenic Children". *Amer. Jour. of Orthopsych.* 17:40, 1947.

[13] Freeman, L., Cameron, J.L. and McGhie, A. *Chronic Schizophrenia.* International Universities Press, N.Y., N.Y., 1958.

[14] Freud, S.: "The Interpretation of Dreams" (I) and (II) in *The Standard Ed. of the Complete Psychological Works* Vols. IV and V. Translated by J. Strachey, Hogarth Press, London, England, 1964.

[15] Bannon, M., Quanbury, A., Cantor, S.: "The Gait of Hypotonic Schizophrenic Children". *Develop. Med. Child Neurol.* 23:770,1981.

[16] Dueck, R., Villafana, P., and Cantor, S.: "The Neuromuscular Functioning of Hypotonic Schizophrenic Children" in preparation.

[17] Freud, S.: "Formulations on the Two Principles of Mental Functioning". *The Standard Ed. of the Complete Psychological Works,* Vol. XII. Translated by J. Strachey, Hogarth Press, London, England, 1964.

[18] Freud, S.: "The Ego and the Id". *The Standard Ed. of the Complete Psychological Works,* Vol. XIX. Translated by J. Strachey, Hogarth Press, London, England, 1964.

[19] Piaget, J.: "Mastery Play" in *Play: Its Role in Development and Evolution* edited by J.S. Bruner, A. Jolly and K. Sylva. Basic Books, Inc., N.Y., N.Y., 1976.

[20] Woodward, Mary: "Piaget's Theory" in *Modern Perspectives in Child Psychiatry* edited by J.G. Howells, Brunner/Mazel, N.Y., N.Y., 1971.

[21] Bender, L.: "The Life Course of Schizophrenic Children". *Biol. Psych.* 2:165, 1970.

[22] Inayatulla, I., Pearce, J., Pezzot-Pearce, T., and Cantor, S.: "Patterns of Functioning on the WISC-R in Hypotonic Schizophrenic Children" in preparation.

[23] Freud, S.: "On Narcissism: An Introduction". *The Standard Ed. of the Complete Psychological Works,* Vol. XIV. Translated by J. Strachey, Hogarth Press, London, England, 1964.

[24] Ireland, D., and Cantor, S. unpublished data.

[25] Wilson, Louise.: *This Stranger My Son.* The New American Library, Inc., N.Y., N.Y., 1969.

[26] Rado, S.: "Schizotypal Organization: Preliminary Report on a Clinical Study of Schizophrenia" in *Psychoanalysis of Behaviour* 2:1, Grune and Stratton, N.Y., N.Y., 1962.

[27] Rubin, T.I.: *Lisa and David; Jordi.* Ballantine Books, a Division of Random House, Inc., N.Y., N.Y., 1962.

[28] Offord, D., and Cross, L.: "Behavioural Antecedents of Adult Schizophrenia. A Review". *Archives of General Psychiatry* 26:267, 1969.

[29] Milani-Comparetti, A. and Gidoni, E.A. "Routine Developmental Examination in Normal and Retarded Children". *Develop. Med. Child Neurol.* 9:631, 1967.

[30] Stern, F.M.: "The Reflex Development of the Infant, A Review". *The Amer. Jour. Occ. Ther.*,XXV(3):155(1971).

[31] Bruininks, R.H.: *Bruininks-Oseretsky Test of Motor Proficiency: Examiner's Manual.* Amer. Guidance Service, Circle Pines, Minn., 1978.

[32] Hinsie, L.E., and Campbell, R.J.: *Psychiatric Dictionary.* Oxford Univ. Press, N.Y., N.Y., 1975.

[33] Kraepelin, E.: *Psychiatrie*, 8th edition. Leipzig:Verlag von Johann Amrosuis Barth, 1913.

[34] Freud, S.: "Infantile Sexuality" and "The Transformations of Puberty" in *The Standard Ed. of the Complete Psychological Works*, Vol. VII. Translated by J. Strachey, Hogarth Press, London, England, 1964.

INDEX